PRAISE FOR

to our health

AND DENISE SOUZA

"My goal was to be proactive with my health and act preventively. I had no health issues just some irritating 'symptoms' I attributed to getting older or just part of life. By identifying and addressing the root issues that involved healing the digestive system, I no longer have bloating or fatigue. I was really excited to see those stubborn few pounds coming off. As a bonus, I saw the end to a troublesome issue with anxiety. I never would have believed some nutritional supplements and a few diet changes would be central to getting my life back! I am achieving wellness and weight loss plus a whole lot more!"

– *Karen Arrizola*

"*To Our Health* is a great resource for anyone looking to improve their diet and their life! The recipes are easy to follow and I love that you can find the ingredients easily. For those with food sensitivities, it's easy to make substitutions however you will hardly need to as the recipes are created to be free of the common allergens. Living free of any particular food can be very challenging. *To Our Health* is an excellent tool to make it easier."

– *Gina P.*

"I just LOVE LOVE LOVE the apple pie green smoothie! Sometimes I feel like I am craving that cinnamon taste with the hint of vanilla! What a fantastic way to be healthy and get in those greens with the morning fruit!

I am also in love with the Cauliflower soup. The rich creamy consistency made me feel like I was getting away with something!"

– Karen Stevenson

"I had been recommended to the GET LEAN program by my physician since every previous attempt at weight loss had failed, including a program where every morsel of food eaten was through a hospital diet clinic. I am thrilled to report that I'm down a total of 33 inches and 24 pounds at the end of four months. A nice surprise was that I never have to feel deprived or hungry."

– Stacie Dye

"Working with Denise and Sue and following their food program was a life changing experience for me. They helped me to develop a healthier relationship with food and I learned that the types of food I put in my body, not counting calories, really makes a difference in losing weight and inches. Working with them, I lost 25 pounds and 31 inches. As a bonus I dropped my cholesterol from 268 to 180 and I was able to stop taking my prescription acid reflux medication!"

– Suzanne Thomas

"The program has changed my whole life as far as eating, cooking, shopping for groceries and eating out is concerned. I eat healthy all the time and continue to feel better. I lost 30 pounds in 5 months and actually want to gain some of it back. I eat 3 big meals and 3-5 snacks a day. I highly recommend this program to anyone who wants to get healthy or to lose weight."

– Carol Moore

"Get Lean!! Really!!! Having been an athlete, an aerobics instructor and now a Massage Therapist, who had been eating for my blood type, I had become very frustrated with the weight gain. My diet was decent. I'm not a junk food eater, so why were my clothes shrinking? Plus, I was feeling super-sluggish and exhausted. Needless to say, I was at the end of my rope. This weight situation seemed hopeless. Then along came Denise and Sue with The Get Lean Program. Muscle testing for sensitivities to foods and supplements, Nutritional Counseling, exercise and group sessions for support to assist in achieving my goals. Once I eliminated the foods that affected me adversely, I began to feel better. The horrible bloating and belching diminished and the inches started to disappear. The Get Lean Goal is for the client to become healthier. During the detoxification process my measurements were taken weekly. During the twelve week program, I lost 15+ inches off my body, but the majority came off my waist. I lost 21 pounds and went from a size 16++++ (they were much too tight, because I refused to buy a larger size) to a size 12. I have remained on my program and now can wear a size 8 skirt and have lost a total of 32 pounds. I am ECSTATIC. I have more energy and stamina than I have had in years! Now, I'm not even tempted to eat "THE WRONG FOODS," because the stiffness, pain, congestion and physical weakness that plagues me afterwards, is no longer worth it! I highly recommend The Get Lean Program to help you to get a new lease on life, too! Thank you so much, Sue and Denise!"

– Brenda C. Money

"I have been struggling with health problems for 10 plus years but the past 2 years were extremely challenging and I was having a hard time functioning on a daily basis. Serious amounts of chronic pain, bloating, fatigue, and stomach issues, breathing problems and anxiety. I found my health was in such a volatile condition every day that most days I couldn't even drive more than a couple of miles away without anxiety about how I was feeling and what would happen if I over did it. I spent numerous times in the hospital in the past few years for various viruses, and neurological problems as well. When I met Denise, I was desperate for help. Though the program was demanding, within a short amount of time I began to do more things without help, I was having less pain, and finally less anxiety! I couldn't believe that eating this way could do so much good. No medication was responsible for the positive change I was experiencing, as far as I'm concerned it was nothing short of a miracle! I am thankful for the divine leading of my creator for taking me to meet such a wonderful, positive person and using her wisdom to put "life" back into my life."

– D.T.

"After receiving no constructive help or guidance from conventional medicine, I decided to try something new and different! I enrolled in the Prescription for Wellness Program with Denise Souza to prevent cancer that had taken the lives of so many of my beloved family members. If I could stave off this terrible disease, I'd like to find a way! My first Bio-electrical Impedance Measurement scan showed several GI issues and kinesiology testing revealed food sensitivities that were causing inflammation in my body and sabotaging my health. Through Denise's 12-week coaching and individualized plan based on whole foods nutrition and a detoxification protocol, I have been able to heal my GI tract, while gaining new energy and losing unwanted weight as an added bonus! Meeting one-on-one with Denise held me accountable and gave me the support I needed to make healthy eating a daily habit. I have benefitted from all the educational seminars, learning from the knowledgeable presenters as well as the participants themselves. I especially value the *To Our Health* cookbook and Healthy Lifestyle Cooking classes that guide me in preparing vegetables and eating nutrient-dense whole foods. It's amazing how you have to learn how to eat all over again as an adult! I highly recommend the Prescription for WELLNESS Program and Healthy Lifestyle Cooking classes for anyone who wants to directly address the cause of their health problems and improve & enhance their overall wellbeing. If given the right nutrition and care, the body is truly a wonder in healing itself!"

– Sheila Jones

"Through the wellness program I have learned to enjoy eating to nourish my body. It feels great to know that I am doing what is best for MY body. By nourishing my body and mind I have found an incredible zest for life and more energy than I ever thought I could have."

– Mandi

to our health

denise souza

May this be a tasty toast to your health. :) Denise

Torchflame Books
An imprint of Light Messages

Denise Souza
BodySymmetry@gmail.com
http://BodySymmetry-Wellness.com
Printed in the United States of America
ISBN: 978-1-61153-031-5

Published by Torchflame Books
books@lightmessages.com
www.lightmessages.com

Cover design by Rachel Souza

Torchflame Books
An imprint of Light Messages

This book is dedicated to those whose paths have crossed mine by God's divine intention to bring me to this very place for this very time.

To Dad, for always telling me to never follow the crowd but rather to be completely different and set apart. Standing apart often means standing alone and being willing to go off the conventional path.

To Mom, for suggesting, with no particular reason, that I read what would be my first "health" book. Her whim ignited my passion.

To Dr. Stephen Driscoll, whose compassion, knowledge and encouragement while treating my family instilled a sense of urgency to share everything I learned from him. He was my transition catalyst from western medicine into holistic care.

To my husband, Jerry and children, Will, Rachel and Craig who have been along for the ride starting as the taste testers with "square chicken" right up until now when they serve as my cheering section, editors, and creative development team.

To Dr. John Schmitt, for his gracious spirit and expertise in developing the programs and teaching me how to implement my knowledge. He was my formation catalyst in providing the platform from which to share my passion.

Thank you

Contents

Acknowledgements	11
A Prescription for Wellness	13
Vegetables	21
Grains	45
Beans	63
Meats	83
Salads	101
Soups	129
Dressings, Sauces, & Dips	149
Smoothies & Beverages	167
Treats... Oh, Yes!	179
21-Day Meal Plan	205
Index	219

Acknowledgements

These recipes are a combination of revised "tried and true" favorites, client creations and just some good old imagination. Compiling the recipes into a book was supposed to be done in a flash and made easy with the cut and paste technique. I will just say I had to frequent my hair stylist for more timely touch ups as the grays were winning the battle! I learned a great deal about things I had no desire to learn regarding computers. I am thrilled the editing and typing is complete and I am proud to share the completed endeavor with you.

I would be completely remiss if I did not take the time to publicly acknowledge those that made this project a success. This was a far larger undertaking then I ever imagined, as these folks can testify to while they helped to keep me sane. Above all I am thankful for the blessing that God has given me through the passion and vision that He has instilled within me to build a wellness community and help clients regain the vibrant health they were created to enjoy. My work is a service foremost unto Him but also to you as we travel together on your journey to wellness.

The Prescription for Wellness Program and the Get Lean Weight Loss Program would not even exist if it were not for my visionary friend, Sue Robinson and the master himself, Dr. John Schmitt. It was Sue's brainchild to approach Dr. Schmitt regarding developing a healthy weight loss program. She envisioned a program that would not be just about weight but one that would mean a new lifestyle, one with vibrant health as the goal. She is my friend, my administrative rock, and co-laborer on this book.

Dr. Schmitt's protocol is the backbone of the programs. His nutritional assessment is the component that sets the programs apart from any other and creates the foundation for the success that follows. He has a servant's heart and a healer's spirit. I have learned invaluable information about nutrition, physiology, and Applied Kineseology. I have also watched the master and gleamed a deeper understanding and appreciation for what it means to be a healer. His expertise, knowledge, and compassion truly set him apart. He views his work as the calling God has placed within him, thus making his patients priority over the business.

My husband and number one supporter and fan, Jerry, gave up countless nights of my company, ate dinners that were a hodge podge of something potentially edible but not really and did it all without complaining. Always the gentleman and often the guinea pig; he patiently allowed me to test out my experimented recipes on his palate. We are looking forward to some evenings together… at least until the next project!

Karen, my amazing friend and "girl Friday," to whom I owe a debt of gratitude and money (if she would only take it!). She has saved the day on countless occasions of total frustration, anger and even tears. She is the one that has taught me things I did not want to know about computer programs. Karen gave up hours and hours to correct my messes. She was always available to me, even staying up late into the night to fix a problem or drive to my house during her lunch hour to work on an issue.

And a thank you to my children for turning the tables on me by NOT doing a task for me but encouraging me to figure it out! Beware; your children remember your tricks! They have always been there for edits, suggestions and most appreciated the encouragement and faith they had in their momma to do a great job!

In Heart Felt Gratitude,

Denise Souza

A Prescription for Wellness

> "Eliminating foods from our diet can greatly improve our quality of health. It can increase our energy, mental clarity, and help our over all well-being. A food intolerance is different than a food allergy. A food allergy is an autoimmune response. A food intolerance can slowly overtime run the immune system down in our Gastro Intestinal tract. It will also compromise our adrenal glands or stress glands. Once the stress glands become stressed they release a chemical called cortisol. This in turn will also suppress the G.I. tract. Eventually more food intolerances will occur due to a distressed G.I. tract. This viscous cycle cannot be stopped unless you eliminate the food the body has become intolerant to. It can take up to 60 days for the body to eliminate all histamines and neurotoxins that are released in response to the food sensitivity. Be patient. The reward is worth the wait!" –Dr. Angela Baylis

Welcome to the program! Whether you are on the GET LEAN Weight Loss Program or the Prescription for Wellness Program, or you simply want to make healthier choices, you have made a very important decision to change your lifestyle by embarking on a journey to wellness. I am humbled by your trust and excited for your future. Wellness is my optimal goal for you through either program. If weight is a concern, it will come into balance as your body heals.

Food sensitivities are one of the cornerstones to success in both programs. Addressing these sensitivities ultimately means you will not be eating those particular foods while on the program and possibly even afterwards. For the vast majority this means the elimination of wheat and dairy, two of the most difficult foods to eliminate with ease; hence the purpose of this cookbook. Each recipe has been created to follow the guidelines of the program, therefore avoiding wheat, dairy, specific spices, certain vegetables and fruits. I hope you enjoy the new experiences, new insight and new foods along your journey.

There is some general information and some guidelines to keep in mind as you use this cookbook and follow the programs, so let's get rolling!

- Eat three meals per day and snack in between. This helps to keep glucose levels balance and avoid highs and lows throughout the day that can cause brain fog and fatigue. It is important to keep your healthy calorie count up with nutrient dense foods. Vegetables have fewer calories per volume than grains and meat. Eat until you are satisfied. You can eat as many vegetables through the day as you like because of their high nutritional benefit, low calorie count, and alkanizing effects.
- Garlic and onions are generally not permitted but are listed in some of the recipes. Various nuts will be on your avoid list but may also be listed in a recipe. For clarification; always adhere to your avoid list and make substitutions or omissions to the recipes accordingly.
- Recipes are only meant to be a guide, not an absolute. Choose within your restrictions but substitute herbs/spices, nuts, vegetables, grains and greens. Also experiment with the amount of certain ingredients, put more of your favorite vegetable or omit an ingredient you don't like.
- Salt is rarely added to the recipes. If you choose to add salt, do so sparingly and use Himalayan salt. For a wonderful salt alternative, fill a salt mill with various dry herbs and spices. Try equal parts of parsley, tarragon, chervil, chives and mint. Or combine oregano,

rosemary, and fennel. No salt is necessary. But if salt is desired, keep it to a minimum, as you will be getting sodium naturally in vegetables and other sources. When adding salt, use ¾ herbs and spices to ¼ Himalayan salt.

- For recipes that call for cooked rice or rice pasta, cook according to package directions with regards to water ratio but omit all oils and salt.
- Purchase herbs and spices from the bulk section for a fraction of the cost.
- The Dressings section has great sauces that will enhance grilled chicken or steamed vegetables. Experiment with the recipes based on what you are mixing them with. For example thicken dressing, turning it into a dip or thin a dip, turning it into a dressing.
- Fresh lemon or lime juice will be a staple flavoring. They can be added to olive oil or sesame oil. But always keep oils to a minimum. Some oils are considered "good fats," but it's one of those areas where too much is no longer good. Some recipes call for oil, but truly good fats are plentiful in nuts, seeds, and avocados. So oils are not necessary for good fat. Sauté with lemon juice, water, and broth rather than oil so the nutritional qualities are not completely destroyed.
- Create new meals by topping rice with leftovers. Vegetables and even some of the salads go great on top of rice. Or start with a bed of greens and top with leftovers. Stacking all of it together is yet another option. Start with greens, top with hot or cold rice then leftovers.
- Agave nectar has generated a bit of controversy. I first learned Amber Agave Nectar results from a higher quality processing, but since doing my own research, I have my doubts regarding its superiority to corn syrup. In such cases, I take the cautious route and use a pure substitute like honey or maple syrup.

- Beverages are limited to water and caffeine free tea only.
    - Water is very important for health and weight loss. Do not drink city water unless you have a quality filter. Refilling jugs from the health food store is acceptable, but the minerals are removed in the reverse osmosis process and are best replaced. You may reuse jugs, but replace the jugs if you are using plastic water jugs of previously purchased distilled spring water, etc. Don't refill jugs more than 2-3 times due to chemicals leaked from plastic. Be sure to use only safe plastic bottles, numbers 2, 4 and 5. A number 7 bottle is good if it specifically says it does not contain BPA. Nalgene bottles are a safe #7 bottle. Drink half your body weight in ounces per day. There are some recipes for flavoring water for those that find drinking plain water difficult.
    - Tea must be labeled 'caffeine free' not 'decaffeinated.' Caffeine free never had caffeine to start with but decaffeinated tea had the caffeine removed, but it is impossible to remove all the caffeine. Caffeine free herbal teas are not advisable because herbs are medicinal.
- Nut flour and grain flours like rice or amaranth can be homemade by blending nuts or grains in a coffee grinder or Vitamix until reaching flour consistency.
- Peanuts are never acceptable due to the presence of aflatoxin; said to be the most potent chemical carcinogen ever discovered.
- Do not use microwaves. Cooking on high is over 400 degrees. Some studies argue the composition of food is altered and nutritional value eliminated.
- VitaMix is a fabulous kitchen appliance ! It makes the best smoothies and will also make nut butters, flours and cook soup.
- Even though a recipe may call for oil, always keep oils to a minimum. Use olive, sesame, or coconut oils.

Proper Food Combining

> "This is what I tell all my patients the first time I see them; 'your nervous system controls everything but your digestive tract rules'. What this means is, if you have any issues with your digestive tract, known or unknown, it will always refer to the area of least resistance in the your body. These symptoms can include joint pain, chronic inflammation, headache pain, chronic sinus, skin issues, fatigue, emotional stress and a full range of other symptoms. So what you eat or drink can dictate your poor health or your vitality. The information in this book can lead you to a more healthy lifestyle."
> –Dr. John Schmitt, DC, Founder of Prescription for Wellness and Get Lean Programs

Proper food combining is extremely important when healing and beneficial for weight loss. Improperly combined foods lead to poor digestion, therefore poor absorption and assimilation of nutrients. The general rule of food combining is: fats and starch go with vegetables, protein goes with vegetables, but starches do not go with protein.

Proper food combining basically goes against the Standard American Died (SAD), no ham or peanut butter sandwich, no chicken stir-fry or spaghetti and meatballs! There are other combination guidelines to adhere to, but the rules are made simple by the coding of each recipe found in this book:

- "P" signifies a recipe is properly combined. There are few "technical combinations that I fudge a bit. Those recipes are rated for those of you who want to be more strict with proper food combining. Apples are something I don't worry much about combining 100% correctly or the treats that include a grain and eggs, such as pancakes.
- "M" is for the maintenance program and is marked accordingly because it will have ingredients that are not on the program and/or are improperly combined.

The GET LEAN Weight Loss Program & The Prescription for Wellness Program

To Our Health! was originally conceived as a cookbook to assist my clients in the GET LEAN Weight Loss Program and the Prescription for Wellness Program. As often happens with meaningful projects, this has grown far beyond my first intentions. But understanding the programs that form the foundation of this cookbook will help you better understand the ultimate goal I have for anyone who picks up this book: to achieve lasting wellness.

In the GET LEAN Weight Loss Program, the goals are to identify root causes that sabotage permanent weight loss efforts, focusing on nutrient levels, food sensitivities, and nutrient dense foods, thus attaining wellness. When balanced, the body naturally drops excess weight. Learn to eat abundantly of tasty foods that assure you of becoming lean for life. GET LEAN is a unique weight loss program with a holistic approach to changing your lifestyle, identifying sabotaging behavior, healing as a goal, encompassing the physical, emotional and physiological aspects of wellness, no product or meals to purchase, centered on whole foods and client education with a team of experts to make goals a reality. Denise holds degrees in Holistic Nutrition and Psychology to be able to coach clients through proper nutritional eating and the emotional aspects and difficulties of permanent weight loss.

The Merriam Webster Dictionary defines prescription as "A written direction or a corrective or therapeutic agent." How would you define your personal prescription for health? The Prescription for Wellness Program writes individualized directions for wellness. Wellness is addressed by focusing on root causes, thus offering the true Prescription for Wellness. The "medicine" in this "script" is food and nutrition. As Hippocrates, the father of medicine, said "Let your food be your medicine and your medicine be your food.

Through education you are empowered to take control of your weight, health and well-being. Changing your lifestyle changes your life. The programs are both designed with the ultimate goal of achieving wellness by addressing root causes and focusing on nutrition. The main difference between the two programs is that clients are weighed and measured in the GET LEAN Program to help them track their progress toward their weight loss goals.

Initial Assessment Process for Participants in the Programs:

- Nutritional Evaluation
- Food Sensitivity Testing
- One-hour Consultation
- Bioelectrical Impedance Measurement Scan

Implementation of 12-Week Program:

- Group or Individual Program Available
- Continual Nutrient Assessment
- Psychological/Emotional Support and Counseling
- 6 Biweekly Coaching Sessions
- Program-specific Guidance on *To Our Health!* Cookbook
- Recipe Conversions
- 2 Bioelectrical Impedance Measurement Scans
- Individualized Wellness Tracking
- Weight and Measurements Tracking
- Educational Information Packet
- 90-Day Commitment Agreement
- Monthly Synergized Living Newsletter Subscription
- Phone and Email Access to Coach

While face-to-face contact is always a bonus in this digital age, clients do not have to live near me to participate in either program. Arrangements can be made for clients living in practically any country around the world.

Vegetables

Vegetables

Veggies… the storehouse for nutrients! While on the program it is generally best to eat the majority of vegetables cooked; this being easier on the digestive process. Vegetables are so versatile; they are wonderful steamed, roasted or grilled. For various textures and presentation, shred, chop or mash, according to personal preference. Always wash vegetables with soap, even if discarding the peel. Bacteria on the peel, can contaminate the flesh as the knife cuts through. Try to increase your cooked vegetable intake to 1 - 2 pounds per day. Once digestive issues have been addressed, aim for 1 pound of cooked vegetables and 1 pound of raw vegetables per day. Remember, vegetables in smoothies and soups count. When eating out, ask for a vegetable to be substituted for the rice or potato, giving you a double order of vegetables. It is best to cook vegetables al dente using any of the methods listed below.

- **Bake:** Average temperature is 325° to 375°
- **Grill:** Average temperature is medium to medium high with very little oil.
- **Oven Roast:** Average temperature is 425° to 450° with very little oil.
- **Sauté:** Average temperature medium to medium high with no oil. Use water, juice or broth.
- **Steam:** Use as little water as possible.

Non-Starchy Vegetables

alfalfa sprouts
artichoke hearts, fresh or frozen
arugula (aromatic salad greens)
asparagus
broccoli
brussels sprouts
bok choy cabbage
cauliflower
celery
collard greens
cucumber
endive
escarole
fennel
green beans
kale
kohlrabi
mustard greens
okra
red leaf (greens)
radishes
rutabaga
romaine lettuce
snow peas
sprouts – all varieties
spring mix (greens)
sugar snap peas
summer squash
spinach
swiss chard
turnips
turnip greens
watercress
water chestnuts
zucchini

Preparation Tips

- Smaller/thinner cuts cook faster
- Dense vegetables cook slower (Ex: Rutabaga)
- High water density vegetables cook faster (Ex: Zucchini)
- Always cook vegetables firm/al dente

Roasted Vegetables

Roasting vegetables enhances sweetness and heightens flavor. Generally, vegetables should be cut, sliced or chopped to approximately the same size. Most importantly, cook high water content vegetables (zucchini) with other high water content vegetables (summer squash). For instance, carrots are dense and have little water compared to zucchini which is not dense and does have a lot of water. Since the zucchini will cook faster than carrots, it should be cooked separately. Carrots are best when partially steamed prior to roasting.

Always roast in single layer; if vegetables are stacked or overlapping they will steam and not roast. Roast in large shallow pan, like a brownie pan, with low sides. Put the pan on the middle rack. If using more than one pan, try to fit them both on the same rack. If this is not possible, put one on bottom and one on middle rack, rotate them after 10 minutes. Shake the pans or flip the vegetables after 10 minutes so they cook evenly. Vegetables in the center of the pan will cook slower, so after 10 minutes move center vegetables to outside.

Coat vegetables with a minimal amount of olive oil. The only reason for the oil is to produce a bit of browning. Vegetables will stick to the pan; do not increase fat content by adding more oil just to prevent sticking. Let them stick, pan can be soaked prior to washing. Vegetables may be coated two ways: put in gallon size baggie with very little olive oil, press air out and seal, hold bag in both hands and move the vegetables about in the bag, put on pan and add spices of choice. Or put vegetables in a large bowl, drizzle very little olive oil and sprinkle spices then toss to coat with your hands, rubbing the oil onto the vegetables. Roast at 425° approximately 10 – 20 minutes. Vegetables should be firmly soft, not over cooked, with browned edges. Vegetables will shrink, so adjust serving portions accordingly.

Vegetables to Roast

Use these vegetables alone or in any combination

asparagus	zucchini
string beans	summer squash
broccoli	butternut squash
cauliflower	garlic and onion
carrot	cabbage
fennel	brussels sprouts

Meal Options

These option work great with leftover vegetables as well

- Eat big bowl of roasted veggies with a salad.
- Add to soup stock for a great soup.
- For creamy soup, puree ½ the vegetables (or more depending on preferred thickness of soup) in a blender and add to broth with remaining vegetables.
- Serve on top of brown rice.
- Serve as pasta topping.
- Add (cold or hot) as salad topping to romaine, baby greens, arugula.
- Cut into thin, lengthwise strips, then use in romaine lettuce roll up with chopped Kalamata olives and sheep/goat feta cheese.
- Serve on a bed of baby spinach, arugula (raw or steamed) or any other greens of choice.

Roasted Root Vegetables (P) (M)

Makes approximately 8 – 9 cups

3 ½ cups sweet potatoes, about 1½ lbs, peeled or unpeeled

3 cups parsnips, about 1 lb

1 ¾ cups turnips, about ½ lb

2 cups winter squash, any variety, about ¾ lb, peeled

3 Tbs. olive oil

1 tsp. natural sweetener of choice (e.g. honey, agave)

½ tsp. sea salt

1 medium red or sweet onion, cut into 8 wedges, do not separate

2 Tbs. chopped fresh parsley

1 Tbs. balsamic vinegar (M) or lemon juice (P)

¼ tsp. freshly ground black pepper

When roasting vegetables, it's important to arrange them in a single layer in the pan to ensure a crisp, golden finish.

Preheat oven to 425°.

Scrub vegetables and cut into chunks. Follow roasting choices found at beginning of Vegetables Section.

Put parsley, vinegar, and pepper in the plastic container. Carefully stir in vegetables (don't get burned!) and coat evenly. Return to pan and bake an additional 15 – 20 minutes until brown and crisp.

Use leftovers for soup or on salad. See "Meal Options" on previous page.

Roasted Whole Okra (P)

Serves 2

18 fresh okra, sliced 1/3 in. thick

1/2 Tbs. extra-virgin olive oil

Preheat oven to 425°. Wash whole okra. Pat dry. Cut off cap and very tip of blossom end and cut into rounds. Place oil and okra slices in a quart size sealable bag. Shake to coat well. Arrange slices in single layer in shallow baking pan or cookie sheet.

Lightly sprinkle with sea salt. Bake for 10 minutes. Stir to brown evenly. Continue baking for 5 – 10 minutes until nicely browned.

Note: For an extra crispy version, cook an additional 5 – 10 minutes.

Roasted okra tends not to be nearly as gummy or slimy as when stewed. And although it's not a problem in this recipe, here's a Dominican Republic tip to eliminate that problem in any recipe where it is a problem:

Place okra in just enough cold water to cover. Squeeze juice of one lime and add to water with rest of lime. Let sit for 10 - 15 minutes, then drain. Pat dry on paper towels.

Grilled Vegetables

Experiment with vegetables of your choice. Directions are basic and used for any vegetable. Always cut larger vegetables into smaller pieces so they cook faster. Use a grilling basket for smaller vegetables. Lightly coat vegetables with olive oil, sprinkle with herbs/spices. Grill on preheated medium grill until tender and browned. These are some vegetable suggestions along with spice and herb suggestions… there are no rules… except to use your imagination!

Good Grilling Vegetables

- zucchini : cut off ends, cut into ⅛ inch lengthwise slices
- summer squash : cut off ends, cut into ⅛ inch lengthwise slices
- broccoli : use florets, peel and cut stem into ⅛ inch lengthwise slices
- cauliflower : use florets
- fennel : discard stalks, trim bottom, cut bulb in half, grill cut side down
- asparagus : use grilling basket to avoid falling through the grill
- onions : slice in rings but do not separate, grill with largest ring down or use grilling basket
- romaine : cut in half lengthwise, grill cut side down
- carrots : first boil until tender but still firm, leave whole
- cabbage: cut in quarters

Spices/Herbs For Grilled Vegetables

rosemary
fennel
basil
oregano thyme
garlic
tarragon
lemon zest
dill

Vegetable Kabobs

1 ½ – 2 cups per serving

Leftovers can be added to chicken broth to make a flavorful soup.

broccoli or cauliflower, large florets
carrot, steamed until fork pierces easily
fennel, small wedges
zucchini or summer squash, large cubes
butternut squash, small cubes
garlic, whole
cabbage, wedges
brussels sprouts, cut in half or steamed lightly, left whole
onion, quartered

Preheat grill to medium. Choose preferred vegetables, cut according to guidelines above. Lightly coat with olive oil and spices of choice. Skewer. Place on hot grill approximately 5 minutes per side or until tender and browned. Serve over big salad or bowl of rice.

Butternut Squash (P)

Serves 2

1 fresh butternut squash (peeled and cubed), or 1 package precut or frozen

fresh lime

Steam squash until soft. Mash with potato masher or fork. When ready to serve, drizzle with fresh lime. If desired, permitted herbs or spices can be added.

Baked Spaghetti Squash (P)

Serves 3 – 4

1 medium spaghetti squash, approximately 2 ¼ lbs

drizzle of olive oil

splash of fresh lemon/lime juice

Preheat oven to 375°. Wash spaghetti squash and cut in half, lengthwise. Scrape out seeds and pulp. Bake, cut side down, for 30 – 40 minutes. Using a hot mitt, hold squash over a bowl and scrape from top to bottom with a fork. Squash will come out like spaghetti noodles. If desired, drizzle with fresh lemon juice.

Spaghetti Squash Ⓟ

Adapted from Dotty Bryn

Serves 2 – 4

1 spaghetti squash

3 tsp. olive oil

1 – 2 Tbs. grated goat cheese or sheep cheese (optional)

¼ cup fresh basil, chopped

2 Tbs. olive tapenade

1 Tbs. pumpkin seeds (optional)

This makes a beautiful fall dish! Top with pumpkins seeds for an extra seasonal touch.

Preheat oven to 350°. Slice squash in half lengthwise. Remove seeds. Place squash cut side up in baking dish with approximately 2 inches of water at the bottom. Cover. Bake until fork tender, approximately 30 minutes. Scoop out squash with a spoon, clean to the skin. Toss loosely with a fork until it appears like spaghetti. Add remaining ingredients in order.

May be served warm as pasta or cold as a salad. You may also add tender asparagus, tender green beans, or roasted pumpkin cubes.

Spaghetti Squash "Pasta" (P)

Serves 4

1 small spaghetti squash

1 small zucchini, sliced in long, thin strips

1 small summer squash, sliced in long, thin strips

basil pesto (in the Dressings, Sauces, & Dips section)

Preheat oven to 350°. Wash spaghetti squash, cut in half, lengthwise. Remove seeds. Place on cooking sheet cut side down. Bake approximately 30 – 40 minutes or until fork pierces skin easily. When cool enough to handle, using an oven mitt, hold squash with one hand, gently pull fork from top to bottom of squash into colander placed in sink. Squash will come out in strings, looking like spaghetti. Let it sit for a few minutes to let water drain out.

While squash is baking, sauté zucchini and summer squash on medium/low. If roasting vegetables, do so before or after spaghetti squash. Roast vegetables according to roasting instructions in Vegetables section.

Rather than draining spaghetti squash in sink; keep spaghetti squash warm by putting the colander inside a stock pan and setting it in the oven, set to 250°. Mix all ingredients. Toss ingredients with approximately 1 Tbs. olive oil and basil pesto, enough to coat.

Zucchini Rollups (P)

Serves 2

2 medium zucchini, sliced, ¼ inch length wise slices

olive oil

spices of choice

stuffing of choice, see below for suggestions

Trim ends of zucchini and discard. Using a sharp, straight edge knife, slice each zucchini lengthwise in uniform ¼ inch slices. It's important not to use large zucchini because they tend to have more seeds, tearing easily when rolled. Medium zucchini is firmer in the center. Using your fingertips (helps to minimize the amount of oil used), lightly coat both side of slices with oil. Sprinkle spices of choice on both sides. Either grill on preheated, medium/high heat until tender (just pliable not soft) or roast zucchini (follow directions for roasting in the Vegetables section).

Stuffing for rollups depends on your imagination. Some suggestions are here, but be creative and experiment. Put about a heaping Tbs. of stuffing at the end of each zucchini slice and roll it up. Place on cookie sheet, end side down, secure with toothpick. Heat in 300° oven or serve at room temperature. It is best to heat the stuffing first if desiring hot rollups because heating after rolling can over cook zucchini. Allow your imagination to soar.

Some fun filling suggestions include:

Seasoned rice
Roasted, steamed or grilled asparagus spears
Sautéed spinach mixed with chopped artichoke hearts
Sheep feta and sautéed spinach

Mediterranean Vegetable Pizza (M)

Serves 2 – 4

For an extra smoky flavor, grill the vegetables rather than sautéing them.

2 medium onions,
thinly sliced lengthwise

3 cloves garlic, chopped

2 colored bell peppers,
thinly sliced lengthwise (red and yellow look great together)

1 medium zucchini, diced

½ – 1 tsp. fresh thyme, crumbled or light dusting of dry herbs (oregano or marjoram may be substituted)

15 Kalamata olives, pitted and halved

½ – 1 cup sheep or goat feta

wheat free pizza or pie shell

Sauté onions on low or medium heat until golden brown and very soft. Add the garlic and sweet peppers, cook until softened, then add the zucchini and cook until tender. Add thyme and olives. Cook for a minute longer. Allow to cool.

Fill pie shell or top pizza crust.

Bake according to package directions. Sprinkle cheese on top for the last 1 – 2 minutes of baking. Serve immediately or enjoy at room temperature. Vegetables may also be grilled rather than sautéed. For more al denté vegetables, slice very thin and top pizza with raw vegetables.

Kohlrabi (P)

Serves 2

2 kohlrabi

olive oil

fresh lemon juice
or lime juice (optional)

Kohlrabi is usually eaten raw, just peeled, sliced and added to a salad. But it's also delicious cooked.

Wash, peel and grate (or slice) kohlrabi, add to sauce pan. Cover with filtered water. Cook on medium heat until tender but not overdone. Drain. Drizzle with olive oil and citrus juice. Serve hot or cold.

Note: These little sputnik-shaped vegetables come in green or purple, and can be eaten raw or cooked. They are related to cabbage. The word kohlrabi is German for cabbage turnip (kohl as in coleslaw, and rübe for turnip), though kohlrabi is more related to cabbage and cauliflower than to root vegetables.

Fennel (P)

Serves 1

1 fennel bulb

Preheat oven to 350°. Trim off stalks, discard. Cut bulb in wedges. Bring water to a boil, place bulbs in pan. Boil about 10 minutes or until fork tender. Drain, place on plate, drizzle with fresh lemon juice, or dressing of choice from Dressings, Sauces & Dips section.

Variations
- *Add raw fennel to any salad.*
- *Mix chopped apple, chopped raw fennel and chopped nuts.*

Baked Apple Fennel (P)

Serves 2

1 bulb fennel

½ apple, cored, chopped

½ tsp. fennel seeds (optional)

⅛ cup walnuts, chopped

Preheat oven to 350°. Trim fennel bulb, discard stalks and slice into thin rings. In baking dish, alternate layers of fennel and apple. Bake approximately 20 - 30 minutes. Top with chopped nuts prior to serving.

If using fennel seeds, mix with fennel and apple. For great optional flavor soak fennel seeds in apple juice for a few hours.

Faux-tatoes (P)

Serves 2 – 4

1 head cauliflower

lemon juice

spices of choice (optional)

drizzle of olive oil

Wash cauliflower. Remove leaves, cut each large floret from stalk, leaving stem. Chop center stalk into small pieces, they take longer to cook then florets. Steam until soft and easily pierced with a fork, about 15 minutes. Place in food processor, or mash by hand until consistency of mashed potatoes. Serve warm. Stir in spices—dried tarragon and fresh parsley are great. Be creative, add spices of choice or diced raw celery after cauliflower is processed; it gives a great crunch. Or cook chopped celery or celery root with cauliflower, following directions above.

Celeriac Sauté (P)

Serves 6

2 cups celeriac (celery root) peeled, shredded or julienned

2 cups celery, sliced

2 Tbs. celery leaves, chopped, (optional)

2 cups cauliflower, cut into florets (optional)

Celeriac is celery root; looks like a whitish, knobby ball. Buy celery that still has some leaves on the stalks. On low/medium heat, sauté celeriac and celery until tender. Add about 2 Tbs. of water to avoid sticking; add more water as needed. Avoid using oil. Add leaves at the end, cook 1 minute longer. Celery contains sodium so salt should not be needed. Drizzle with lemon juice if desired. Celeriac and celery may also be steamed and mashed, just like mashed potatoes.

If using cauliflower, steam first then add to sautéed celeriac and celery, leaving them all chunky or mash all ingredients.

Cheesy Cauliflower (P)

Serves 3 – 4

1 head cauliflower

2 cloves garlic

juice from ½ lemon

olive oil

aged goat cheese or pecorino (sheep), finely grated

Preheat oven to 400°. Cut cauliflower into florets. Wet finger tips with olive oil; rub cauliflower florets. Place in a large oven-proof baking dish, spreading in a single layer. Peel and coarsely mince garlic. Mix with lemon juice. Sprinkle mixture over cauliflower.

Bake 25 – 30 minutes or until lightly browned. Fork tines should easily pierce floret when done. Sprinkle with goat cheese. Return to oven until cheese is melted. Serve immediately.

Lemony Nutty Green Beans (P)

Serves 2

1 ½ lbs fresh green beans, trimmed,
cut into ½ in. pieces, or frozen and defrosted

½ cup nuts

2 Tbs. parsley, chopped

1 ½ tsp. lemon zest

2 tsp. olive oil

Roasting beans and tossing with remaining ingredients is a tasty alternative.

Steam beans until tender, about 7 minutes. Drain, transfer beans to bowl. Toss with the remaining ingredients. Cilantro may be substituted for parsley.

Zesty Asparagus (P)

Serves 2

1 lb fresh asparagus (approximately 1 bunch)

1 tsp. lemon zest, preferably organic
or be sure to use soap to wash the peel

2 Tbs. aged goat cheese, finely grated

Mix lemon zest, olive oil and goat cheese in a serving bowl. Wash asparagus. Cut off tough portion (white) on bottom of each stalk. Cut asparagus diagonally into 2-inch sections. Bring approximately 1 inch of water to boiling.

Add cut asparagus. Cover. Steam approximately 3 – 5 minutes, until just cooked (al denté). While hot, with lemon zest. Top with cheese and serve.

Steamed Pea Pods (P)

Serves 2 – 3

1 ½ cups sugar snap peas per serving

fresh lemon

spices of choice

De-string pea pods but do not shuck peas. Steam. Drain. Drizzle juice to taste. Sprinkle with spice mix.

A big bowl of these makes a great lunch!

Peas and Lettuce (P)

Serves 4

3 cups fresh or frozen peas

1 head romaine lettuce, coarsely chopped (or other lettuce of choice)

3 cloves garlic, minced

¼ tsp. dried basil

¼ tsp. dried thyme

¾ cup filtered water

Sauté garlic in ¼ tsp. olive oil for 1 minute on low heat. Add vegetables. Sauté, without water, until the lettuce begins to wilt. Continue cooking on low/medium heat until all vegetables are cooked. If necessary add small amounts of water to prevent sticking. May be served as a side dish or over rice.

Sautéed Escarole (P)

Serves 4

1 tsp. olive oil

1 Tbs. garlic, sliced

1 large head escarole, about 1 lb

lemon juice (optional)

If desired, substitute rosemary or fennel for garlic.

In large skillet, add garlic and 1 tsp. olive oil. Sauté on low/medium about 1 minute. Add escarole, cook, tossing as it cooks. It should give off its own water so there is no need to add more oil. If it starts to stick, add a few drops of water. Optional: drizzle with lemon juice.

Creamed Kale (P)

Serves 4

2 bunches kale

1 cup raw nuts or 3 – 4 Tbs. raw nut butter
(cashew, pine nut, sunflower seed or pumpkin seed)

1 cup nut milk or rice milk

4 Tbs. organic onion flakes (if permitted), toasted if you can find them

1 Tbs. seasoning of choice such as tarragon, if not using onion flakes.

Tear leaves from stems. Steam 10 – 15 minutes, until just soft (al denté). Meanwhile, place remaining ingredients in high-powered blender, blending until smooth. Place cooked kale in colander, press to remove excess water. Coarsely chop kale, mix with cream sauce.

Swiss Chard Pie (P)

Serves 4 - 6

1 large bunch swiss chard

½ cup swiss chard stalks, cut in thin slices

3 whole eggs, beaten (may substitute 6 whites or 6 yolks)

1 small onion, thinly sliced, enough to cover top

thin topping goat/sheep cheese

In the place of swiss chard, you may substitute approximately 8 ounces of spinach.

Preheat oven to 350°.

Wash swiss chard, paying close attention to cleaning both sides. Remove leaves from stem, saving the two largest stalks to be used for topping. Wilt leaves using vegetable steamer or sauté in pan. If sautéing, do not add oil, let it wilt in its own juice. Transfer to lightly oiled 9-inch glass pie plate.

Pour beaten eggs over swiss chard. Sprinkle top with chard stalks which have been thinly sliced. End with sprinkling of grated cheese.

Bake 25 – 30 minutes, until egg is set and top is lightly browned. Eat hot or cold.

Note: Omit cheese for proper food combining.

Collard Greens Minera (P)

Serves 2

1 bunch collard greens

3 slices uncooked turkey bacon, chopped

fresh lime or lemon, to taste

Wash and cut collard leaves in half lengthwise. Remove center rib and bottom stem from each leaf. Stack several leaves. Roll tightly, into a cigar shape. With sharp knife, cut across stack into very thin ⅛ inch slices or shreds resembling thin ribbons.

Cook bacon in large skillet on medium heat, stirring, until half cooked. Add collards, tossing to coat, cook until collards are bright green and bacon is crisp, about 3 minutes. Drizzle with citrus juice. Top with shredded pecorino cheese if desired.

Arugula Frittata (P)

Serves 1

1 cup arugula or other greens

2 eggs (or egg whites)

Toasted onion, to taste

Garlic powder, to taste

Sauté arugula or other greens, sprinkle with toasted onion and garlic powder, add 2 eggs (or egg whites) over greens, cover and cook on low until egg is set.

Grains

Grains

Enjoy alternating the grains in these recipes. While on the program, brown rice is usually the most often permitted, but don't be nervous about experimenting. Although not well known, Quinoa is an ancient grain, high in protein and is wonderful with Hijike seaweed. Rice is not a grain but actually a grass. Buckwheat is actually a completely separate grain and not in the wheat family. And corn is a grain, not a vegetable.

For rice pasta, Tinkyada is a good brand found in health food stores. Trader Joe's has their brand and it is tasty as well. When purchasing rice pasta, always go with brown rice. There are white rice versions, but those are void of nutrition and not part of the program. For quickie meals, mix cooked rice with left over vegetables or soup. Defrost frozen vegetables and mix with cooked rice, add a splash of lemon juice. Avocado mashed with lemon juice is great for topping tortilla chips, fast and easy.

Leftover grains tend to dry out a bit. When reheating leftovers, add water or broth to the pan, or add lemon juice when serving. It's fun to even change up the leftovers by topping with a sauce or dressing.

Gluten Free Grains

Brown Rice
Buckwheat
Quinoa
Wild Rice
Amaranth
Teff
Rice Pasta
Oats (controversial)

Cooking Times for Grains

Grain (1 cup)	*Water*	*Cooking Time*
Amaranth	2 cups	20 minutes
Barley (pearl)	3 cups	30 minutes
Basmati rice	1 ¾ cups	15 - 20 minutes
Brown rice (long-grain)	2 cups	30 minutes
Brown rice (short- or medium-grain)	3 cups	45 minutes
Wild rice	3 ¾ cups	45 minutes
Buckwheat	2 cups	20 minutes
Millet	2 cups	30 minutes
Quinoa	2 cups	15 minutes
Quinoa (alternative)*	2 cups	5 minutes

Combine grains and water in pan. Bring to a boil, cover. Reduce heat to low, simmer until tender. When grains are cooked, all liquid will be absorbed into the grain. For every 1 cup of uncooked grain, the average yield is about 2-3 cups of cooked grain. Follow directions on the package, but omit added salt or fats. Let cooked grains stand, covered, for 5 minutes. Fluff with a fork before serving.

*For Quinoa alternative, soak in filtered water approximately 1 – 2 hours. Drain soaking water. Add ⅛ cup water, cover. Cook over medium heat.

Asian Grain (P)

Serves 2

> *Grains and seaweeds may be hot or cold but all other ingredients need to be cold or room temperature.*

2 cups cooked quinoa or brown rice
1 avocado, cubed
1 medium carrot, grated
3 Tbs. cucumber, chopped
1 Tbs. raw sesame seed
1 Nori sheet, torn into ½ in. pieces
12 drops sesame oil
2 tsp. fresh lime juice
other seaweeds of choice for extra minerals and texture, rehydrated

In bowl, toss all ingredients except avocado. Add sesame oil and lime juice to taste. Top with avocado—tossing it in can make it mushy.

If rehydrating the seaweed, add a bit of the water to moisten the quinoa if desired. Leftover quinoa will dry out a bit. Reserve some seaweed water to remoisten or add plain water. Another splash of lime juice brings out the flavor in leftovers as well.

Mock Fried Rice (P)

Serves 4

2 cups cooked brown rice

½ cabbage, shredded (green, Napa, or mixed)

1 carrot, shredded

1 cup peas

½ onion, sliced thinly

fresh lemon juice

sesame oil to taste

garlic

black sesame seeds

This is a quick, versatile dish. Fresh or frozen vegetables. For fresh vegetables, sauté in batches on medium-low heat, so they 'sweat' in their own juices. If they begin to stick, add water, lemon juice or broth. Or roast vegetables by following directions for roasting vegetables in the Vegetables section. If using frozen vegetables, heat in pan or in oven. When cooked, sprinkle with sesame oil and lemon juice.

When rice is cooked, drizzle a few drops of sesame oil. Use raw sesame oil rather than toasted. It's strong, so use only a few drops at a time, tasting as you go. Add a few squeezes of lemon juice. Mix rice well. Add vegetables. Mix well again. Sprinkle sesame seeds prior to serving.

Hijiki with Rice (P)

Serves 4 – 6

½ cup cooked brown rice

2 ½ Tbs. dried Hijiki
(substitute with other seaweed if desired)

1 lb frozen edamame, defrosted (non GMO)

1 tsp. sesame oil (raw, not toasted)

⅛ cup fresh lemon juice

1 Tbs. accepted sweetener

½ daikon radish, about the size of a large carrot, shredded

1 large carrot, shredded

4 handfuls baby spinach

Rehydrate hijiki in bowl of hot water approximately 20 minutes. It will double in volume so use a big enough bowl. Make dressing: mix oil, sweetener, lemon juice and set aside. Use a vegetable peeler to peel carrot and daikon into strips or cut into matchsticks or shred.

In large bowl, toss greens, hijiki, carrot, daikon and edamame. Add dressing slowly, just enough to coat vegetables lightly. Mix with hot rice. If you don't prefer mixing hot and cold ingredients, cook rice ahead and refrigerate to be added cold. Omitting the rice, makes a great salad.

Brown Rice with Asparagus (P)

Serves 2

1 cup cooked brown rice

1 bunch asparagus, cut diagonally into 1 in. pieces

⅓ English cucumber, chopped

1 Tbs. fresh mint, chopped

1 Tbs. fresh cilantro, chopped

1 lemon or lime

Steam chopped asparagus until al dente' (tender but firm). Meanwhile, chop cucumber. Mix cucumbers with herbs in a large bowl. Drain asparagus. Add to bowl. Add cooked rice. Drizzle juice of ½ – 1 fresh lemon or lime, depending on personal taste. If mixture is too dry, put another ⅛ – ¼ cucumber in blender and add to moisten. Peel the cucumber if you don't want "green" rice.

Serve hot or cold.

As a variation, you can omit herbs and top with a sauce from the Dressings, Sauces, & Dips section.

Grilled Vegetables with Rice (P)

Serves 2

1 cup uncooked brown rice

2 large zucchini or summer squash

1 tsp. olive oil

dried spices/herbs of choice:
rosemary, fennel, basil, oregano, thyme, etc

fresh lemon or lime

2 large handfuls arugula, baby spinach or mixed greens

Cut ends of squash. Cut squash into ⅛ inch lengthwise slices. Coat fingertips with oil and coat squash on both sides. Sprinkle with spices/herbs of choice. Set aside. Drizzle a small amount of olive oil and squeeze ½ lime or ¼ lemon into cooked rice, mix. Approximately 10 minutes before rice is finished, grill squash on medium heat until tender but do not overcook. Cook approximately 3 minutes per side. Cut squash and mix with rice.

Options:
If using greens; layer greens on dinner plate, with hot rice on top then hot squash.
Mix with Artichoke Sauce or Avo-choke Sauce in Dressings section.

Green Rice (P)

Serves 2

> *Adjust quantities to personal preference.*

2 cups cooked brown rice

½ - 1 small zucchini squash, minced

1 ½ cups fresh spinach, minced

¼ cup fresh basil, minced

⅛ cup fresh parsley, minced

1 clove garlic, minced

1 Tbs. extra virgin olive oil

1 - 2 Tbs. fresh lemon juice or raw apple cider vinegar (vinegar not permitted on program)

Put cooked rice in bowl. Gently mix in all raw vegetables. Drizzle a little olive oil and vinegar or lemon juice to taste. Vegetables can be mixed while rice is hot, so vegetables wilt slightly. Leftovers are best cold or at room temperature. To reheat, add a bit of water to sauce pan, add rice mixture, heat on low, stirring often.

Makes a great picnic lunch!

Zippy Zucchini Rice (P)

Serves 2

1 cup uncooked rice, any variety

2 medium zucchini, shredded

4 Tbs. fresh basil, chopped

4 Tbs. fresh mint, chopped

½ cup green peas (thawed frozen or cooked fresh peas)

½ avocado, sliced or cubed

cilantro, chopped (optional)

Dressing:

juice of ½ lemon (approx. 1 Tbs.)

½ tsp. dried oregano

½ English cucumber, peeled, blended until liquid

Combine zucchini, basil, mint, peas and set aside. Blend together lemon juice, blended cucumber, and oregano. Combine hot rice, zucchini mixture and dressing. Top with avocado. Enjoy cilantro to taste.

Rice Stuffed Cabbage Leaves (P)

Makes approximately 25-30 rolls

1 large green cabbage or collard greens

4 cups cooked brown rice

1 large onion, finely chopped

1 Tbs. fresh mint, finely chopped

5 cloves garlic, minced

⅔ cup zucchini, finely chopped

½ cup fresh parsley, finely chopped

1 cup filtered water (approximately)

juice of 1 lemon (about 4 Tbs.)

Cut out core of cabbage. Stick a large fork into center. Bring large pot of filtered water to a boil. Immerse cabbage, leaving fork in place. When outer leaves turn bright green, remove from pan. Using fork, gently peel away softened leaves. Return to pot. Repeat until all cabbage leaves have been removed.

If using collard greens, blanch leaves in hot water until softened and darker green. Gently shave down thick stems if desired. Cut very large leaves in half.

To make stuffing mix: sauté onion, garlic, and zucchini. Add herbs and spices. Set aside.

To make rolls, fill leaf with stuffing. Place stuffing 1 inch from thick end of cabbage leaf. Fold bottom over filling, fold sides in, roll up.

(Recipe continued on next page.)

Preheat oven to 350°. In large baking dish, place rolls closely together, seam side down. Layer if necessary. Add lemon juice to enough water to cover bottom of dish. Bake uncovered 30 minutes. May also be eaten at room temperature.

Optional: Drizzle with Creamy Herb dressing from Dressings, Sauces, & Dips section when serving.

Cold Rice Noodle Salad (P)

Serves 4

1 bag 16 ounce frozen peas, defrosted

1 jar artichoke hearts, jarred in water or 8 frozen artichoke hearts, chopped

1 English cucumber, diced

juice 1 fresh lemon

1 tsp. sesame oil

1 small section clear (cellophane) rice noodles, or other rice pasta

1 Tbs. black sesame seeds

fresh cilantro, optional for garnish

You may also add shredded carrots or sliced avocado

Cook pasta according to directions, drizzle with sesame oil. Place in refrigerator to cool. Mix remaining ingredients in bowl. Combine noodles and vegetables. If not eating immediately, do not add lemon juice or oil until ready to serve. Lemon juice looses flavor after sitting in refrigerator as does oil; so it is always best to dress a salad prior to eating. Garnish with sesame seeds and fresh cilantro. Clear rice noodles come in various sizes but they are usually packaged in bundles within a package, so use one bundle.

Pasta with Fresh Avocado Sauce (P)

Serves 2

8 ounce package cooked, brown rice pasta

2 ripe avocados

¼ cup unsweetened rice milk, or nut milk, or water

½ cup fresh basil, chopped

juice ½ fresh lemon (optional)

Cook pasta according to package directions. Drain. While pasta is cooking, slice avocado around center lengthwise, twist to separate the halves. Holding one half in the palm of your hand or lay it on a cutting board. With a sharp, straight edge knife hit the pit so knife lodges in the pit. Twist knife to remove nut. Using a spoon, scoop out flesh. Mash with fork.

Heat rice milk on low. Remove from heat, add mashed avocado and lemon juice (if using) to hot milk. Put hot pasta in bowl, add avocado sauce, and fresh basil. Stir to combine.

Sweet Potato (or Yam) Biscuits Ⓜ

Makes 8 – 12 biscuits

If you've tried converting recipes to gluten free, you know that most recipes call for a small amount of xanthan gum to replace the gluten (½ tsp. to 1 cup brown rice flour). In this recipe there's a choice between xanthan gum *or* tapioca flour.

1 cup sweet potatoes or yams, cooked and mashed

⅓ cup butter, melted

1 egg, beaten

1 cup brown rice flour

2 Tbs. tapioca starch (or ½ tsp. xanthan gum + 1 Tbs. brown rice flour)

2 tsp. aluminum-free baking powder

½ tsp. sea salt

Preheat oven to 350°.

Mix first three wet ingredients separately from remaining dry ingredients. Then combine, mixing thoroughly. Spoon a heaping tablespoon (or use a small ice cream scoop) onto cookie sheet. Bake for 35 – 40 minutes until nicely browned.

Gluten-Free Pancakes (M)

by Diane Timoney

Serves 4 – 6

Dry ingredients:

- 2 cups brown rice flour
- 3 Tbs. tapioca starch
- ⅔ cup ground hemp seed
- 1 Tbs. aluminum-free baking powder
- 1 tsp. baking soda
- ½ tsp. salt

Liquid ingredients:

- 1 Tbs. permitted liquid sweetener
- 2 eggs (may substitute 4 yolks or 4 whites), beaten
- ¼ cup unsweetened applesauce, cinnamon flavored preferred
- 2 cups water or rice milk

Beat eggs using a wire whip or hand mixer. Mix dry and liquid ingredients separately. Quickly fold dry and liquid ingredients together. Spoon onto preheated skillet or griddle. When bubbles form, flip to cook other side until golden brown.

Almond Flour Pancakes (M)

Serves 4 – 6

1 cup almond flour (almond meal)

½ tsp. aluminum-free baking powder

⅛ tsp. salt

2 Tbs. extra virgin olive oil

2 eggs (may substitute 4 yolks or 4 whites)

¼ cup filtered water

1 Tbs. permitted liquid sweetener

Preheat skillet or griddle. Mix ingredients together. Grill as you would other pancakes. The only real difference is they won't "bubble" on top the same way as regular pancakes. Flip when underside is brown.

Rolled Oats Hot Cereal (M)

Serves 1

½ cup rolled oats (not instant)

1 cup unsweetened rice or nut milk

½ cup unpeeled apple, peach or pear, chopped (optional)

permitted sweetener (optional)

⅛ cup permitted nuts, chopped

Adding fruit could be a problem for those following strict food combining.

Heat rice milk in small pan (hot, not boiling). Transfer to cereal bowl. Stir in oatmeal. Let set 2 – 3 minutes or until liquid is absorbed. Top with nuts and fruit.

Beans

Beans

WOW, BEANS ARE ONE OF MY FAVORITE THINGS TO EXPERIMENT WITH. They are incredibly versatile, lending themselves to simple, hearty soups and creamy dips to sweet, chocolaty brownies! No kidding, brownies! Beans can be so much fun that I put them in their very own chapter. There is only one recipe here that calls for dried beans. I have a friend who cooks dried beans on a regular basis with no complaints to time or effort. But I still have not come around to that idea and reach for the can. Beans are one of only three things I will even purchase in a can. As always, read the ingredients to make sure there is minimal salt (salt should not exceed double the calories) and no preservatives. To make a fast, easy soup; simply add broth to leftovers and if you need a bit more substance add some veggies or a grain. One of my favorite things is a bean salad; I eat them as is or tossed with chopped greens or mixed with hot or cold rice. Beans are a healthy and easy way to adjust to less animal protein in your diet. Beans are a power house of fiber, protein, vitamins and minerals. When a salad isn't enough to fill you, top it with beans. Add beans to various soups. It is so easy to be creative with beans. Like all the recipes, simply think of you taste preferences and mix and match ingredients! This is probably the easiest and most fun chapter to experiment with on ingredients. Be bold and brave, switch out the types of beans in the recipes and create your own version. Don't be locked into a recipe, mine or any other—think outside the box (or the can)!

Common Types of Beans

white beans
black beans
pinto beans
kidney beans
lima beans
chickpeas
black eyed peas
cannellini beans

Preparation Tips

- When using dry beans, soak the beans for at least 4 hours to help remove toxins and facilitate digestion.
- Slow cooking dry beans in a crock pot helps ensure a creamy texture.
- To easily thicken soups, blend some of the beans from the recipe with some of the broth from the soup.
- Always cook beans until they are soft.

Creamy White Bean Soup Ⓜ

Serves 2 – 4

2 cups dried white beans, great northern or cannellini

6 cups water or organic chicken broth

1 medium onion, chopped

6 cloves garlic, chopped

1 bay leaf

olive oil (optional)

Optional Toppings

fresh rosemary, chopped

scallions, chopped

sun dried tomatoes, diced

fresh, roasted grape tomatoes seasoned with garlic powder

Rinse beans thoroughly. In crock pot add beans, onion, garlic, and bay leaf. Cover and cook on low for about 8 hours, or until beans are tender. Remove the bay leaf. Blend all the soup in batches in a blender or food processor and return to pan. Or blend some and leave some beans whole. Ladle into bowls. Drizzle with the olive oil. Garnish with your selection of toppings.

Kickin' Black Bean Soup Ⓜ

Serves 4 – 6

2 cans (15 oz) black beans, drained

1 large onion, chopped

1 medium sized carrot, chopped

1 small red bell pepper, seeded and minced

3 cloves garlic, minced

1 small, fresh hot chile, seeded and minced

1 can (15 oz) diced tomatoes with liquid

6 cups low sodium vegetable broth, organic chicken broth or water

1 tsp. dried oregano

1 tsp. ground cumin

¼ tsp. cayenne (optional)

2 Tbs. fresh cilantro, minced, for garnish (optional)

Serving Suggestions

Add grated pecorino Romano or sheep feta cheese on top of each bowl

Squeeze fresh lime juice into each bowl just before serving.

Garnish with chopped scallions

If you prefer a milder taste, omit the chile and/or cayenne. Sauté onion, carrot, bell pepper, garlic and chile on low so they sweat and cook in their own juices. If it starts to stick add water or broth. Cover and cook until softened. Drain the juice from the tomatoes into the pan and dice the tomatoes very small then add to the pan. Simmer for 30 minutes or until all vegetables are soft. Carefully transfer 2 cups of soup to a blender or food processor. If using a blender be very careful to hold the lid on but lift the center piece up once it is going to let steam escape. Process until smooth then return to pan. Add water or broth if it is too thick. Adjust the seasonings. Garnish with cilantro.

White Bean with Escarole Soup (M)

Serves 2

1 can white, cannellini or navy beans, do not drain

4 cloves garlic, minced

1 large leek stalk, white portion with ¼ of green portion, sliced thin

1 head of fresh escarole, about 1 pound

16 oz organic chicken broth

3 Tbs. olive oil

Remove the end of the leek and one outer layer, just as you would for a scallion. Slice and break into rings, rinse well as they are very sandy. Wash escarole and chop. Sauté escarole, garlic and leek in oil until they begin to soften. Add beans with liquid, broth and simmer, covered, on low until heated through.

Italian White Bean Soup Ⓜ

Serves 2

1 can white, cannellini or navy beans, do not drain

1 large leek stalk, white portion with ¼ of green portion, sliced thin

1 head of fresh escarole, about 1 pound

½ cup chopped carrots

½ cup chopped celery

½ cup cherry tomatoes

2 tsp. Italian seasoning

1 sprig fresh rosemary

4 cloves garlic, minced

3 Tbs. olive oil

8 oz organic chicken broth

1 can (15 oz) chopped tomatoes

Remove the end of the leek and one outer layer, just as you would for a scallion. Slice and break into rings, rinse well as they are very sandy. Wash escarole and chop. Sauté fresh vegetables, Italian seasoning, garlic, and rosemary in oil until they begin to soften. Add beans with liquid, broth, and tomatoes. Simmer covered on low until heated through.

Garlicky Beans and Greens Ⓜ

Serves 2 – 3

This recipe calls for more oil then I usually suggest, but it makes a big difference in this recipe.

Substitute other spices such as 1 Tbs. fennel seeds or ½ Tbs. rosemary.

1 can cannellini beans,
navy beans may be substituted

1 leek or 1 bunch of scallions, sliced

10 cloves of garlic, chopped

2 bunches chard, or other greens, chopped

7 – 7 Tbs. of olive oil

black pepper

Pecorino Romano cheese, shredded (optional)

Drain the beans and reserve the liquid. If using the leek, slice and break apart the rings. Rinse well as they are very sandy; set aside. In pan, add 5 cloves of garlic, leeks and fresh ground pepper with about 3 – 4 Tbs. of olive oil, simmer on low for about 5 minutes. Add drained beans and let cook on low while preparing the greens; stir periodically to prevent sticking. Simmering for 30 minutes allows the garlic flavor to permeate the beans beautifully.

Wash and cut greens and set aside. In a separate larger pan (large enough to hold all the greens), add 2 – 3 Tbs. of olive oil and 5 cloves of chopped garlic; sauté on low to flavor the oil, about 3 – 5 minutes; do not brown. Set aside. Add chopped greens to pan and sauté on medium heat. There is no need for more oil. The greens will sweat and steam in their own water. Arugula tends to be more dry, so adding a little water may be necessary. Continuously toss until almost completely wilted then add garlic oil and continue cooking, tossing, until garlic is soft and greens are completely wilted. *(Recipe continued on next page.)*

Plate the greens and top with beans and cheese, if using.

Use leftovers or to make soup; simply add all cooked ingredients to chicken or vegetable broth.

Serving Suggestions:

- Layer: fresh arugula or cooked arugula then hot, brown rice then hot beans.
- Cut romaine hearts lengthwise one time, brush a little olive oil on the cut side, broil or grill (they will burn easily) until leaves are browned around the edges. Then top with bean mixture (without arugula), sprinkle with grated Pecorino Romano cheese (optional).
- Green options: 16 oz arugula or 2 bunches of kale or collard greens.
- Omit greens and enjoy beans and rice together.

White Bean Chili (M)

Serves 3 – 4

1 onion, chopped

2 cans white beans, cannellini or northern, do not drain

16 oz organic chicken broth

1 cup organic fresh or frozen corn

1 can green chilies, chopped

2 tsp. cumin

1 Tbs. oregano

1 tsp. chili powder

3 scallions, chopped for garnish (optional)

10 black olives, chopped for garnish (optional)

Sauté onion on low/medium so it will sweat and cook in its own juice. In saucepan, add remaining ingredients except scallions and olives. Cook on medium until bubbling then reduce to simmer. Simmer, uncovered for 20 – 30 minutes. Stir periodically to prevent sticking. If chili still has too much liquid, mash with potato masher until you reach the desired consistency.

This recipe tastes best the next day once the ingredients have had time to meld their flavors. Garnish with scallions and/or olives at time of serving.

Great served with polenta and avocado!

Bean Chili and Sweet Potatoes Ⓜ

Serves 4 – 6

1 can black beans, drained

1 can adzuki beans, drained

1 can white kidney beans, drained

1 can (28 oz) chopped tomatoes, drained
(Fire roasted are great!)

2 tsp. cumin

1 Tbs. chili powder

2 cups chunky salsa or picante sauce, mild or medium

2 medium sweet potatoes, peeled and cubed

1 bunch scallions, sliced

1 bunch fresh cilantro (optional)

Roast or steam sweet potatoes until al dente and set aside.

Combine remaining ingredients and cook on medium for 15 – 20 minutes, lower heat if chili begins to stick. Chili will thicken as it cooks down. If it needs to be thicker, mash some of the bean mixture using a fork. Add the potatoes when the chili is done. If using cilantro, add 1 cup to the chili as it cooks and add more for garnish when serving.

Serving Variations:

- Garnish with sliced avocado or a spoonful of guacamole
- Serve on top of sliced, pre-made polenta
- Serve on a bed of raw lettuce, arugula, spinach or mixed greens with ranch dressing drizzled on greens, then add chili.

- Cut romaine heart in half lengthwise, lightly brush with olive oil and broil until ends wilt and brown. Place on dinner plate, drizzle with Ranch dressing, cover with chili and garnish with cilantro or a drizzle of dressing.
- Add organic corn and/or black olives.
- Garnish with scallions, sliced.
- Mix with cooked brown rice.
- Use in a brown rice tortilla skin.
- Add leftovers to broth and make soup.

Versatile Southwestern Rice (M) (P)

Serves 4

2 cups cooked brown rice
1 can black or pinto beans, drained
1 – 2 cups salsa of choice (such as Pace picante, mild or a black bean salsa) (M)
1 cup fresh cilantro chopped
1 can (16 oz) black olives (chop half)
1 cup fresh or frozen corn
1 can green chilies (M)
1 bunch of scallions, sliced
1 – 2 cups fresh tomatoes, chopped
1 – 2 fresh limes, squeezed for juice
Pecorino Romano or other sheep/goat cheese as garnish, optional

Cook rice according to package instructions. Warm the beans or leave at room temperature.

(Recipe continued on next page.)

In a bowl, combine remaining ingredients except cheese. When rice is cooked and still very hot add all ingredients and mix. Corn, tomatoes, cilantro and scallions will remain raw for a stronger flavor. Adjust measurements and omit ingredients according to personal taste.

This dish acts as a base for other meals. Cook extra and use leftovers to:

- stuff bell peppers or poblano peppers and bake
- stuff tomatoes
- serve on a bed of arugula or baby spinach that was tossed in lime and olive oil
- add leftovers to broth for a quick soup
- wrap in brown rice tortilla skin to make a burrito
- use as a topping for polenta
- serve with avocado

Marinated Bean Salads (P) (M)

The following recipes all follow the same process. Marinate beans for at least one hour. The flavor grows more intense the longer they marinate. To marinate, place drained beans in a jar or leak proof container. Fill jar until half the beans are covered. Depending on how long you decide to marinate the beans, flip the jar at the half-way point. Drain the beans and reserve the marinade. Add the beans and remaining ingredients in bowl and toss with a little remaining marinade if needed. If you are on a maintenance plan and choose to use flavored vinegars, Perel is a fantastic choice free of preservatives and nitrates. Be daring and mix up the beans and add ingredients of your own choosing, mix the ingredients between these recipes, or omit what you don't like.

These recipes are also great when served over a bed of greens or added to cooked rice.

White Bean Artichoke Salad

1 can white beans or chickpeas

flavored vinegar of choice (M) or fresh lemon juice (P)

½ cup artichoke hearts, sliced, use frozen or jarred in water only

¼ cup black olives, sliced, preferably Kalamata, or green olives

¼ – ½ cup celery, sliced

¼ cup sun dried tomatoes in oil, chopped or reconstitute the dry tomatoes

2 Tbs. sweet onion, minced (optional, not good if storing for more than a day)

Pecorino Romano or sheep or goat feta cheese (optional)

fresh basil sliced (optional)

Black Eyed Pea and Cucumber Salad

1 can black eyed peas

3 lemons, squeezed

2 medium stalks celery, chopped

⅛ cup black olives, sliced

⅛ cup Kalamata olives, sliced

1 small English cucumber, diced

1 cup organic raw corn or ⅔ cup frozen, defrosted

1 medium tomato, chopped Ⓜ

⅛ cup sun dried tomatoes in oil, chopped

¼ cup sheep or goat feta cheese, optional

fresh basil, chopped, optional

Black Bean and Corn Salad

1 can black beans

3 lemons, squeezed and mixed with 2 tsp. ground cumin Ⓜ

a few drops of hot sauce can be optionally added to the marinate Ⓜ

1 cup organic raw corn or ⅔ cup frozen, defrosted

2 – 3 scallions, chopped

1 medium sweet potato, roasted and cut into small cubes

8 black olives, chopped

1 bunch fresh cilantro, chopped (about 1 cup)

1 avocado, chopped
(it will oxidize, so eat immediately after chopping)

1 small clove garlic, minced

Bean Dips (P) (M)

Hummus is a bean dip made with chickpeas and tahini and can be found in the grocery store and Mediterranean delis. Other bean dips can be purchased at specialty stores and the Southwestern section of grocery stores. Most food purchased this way have far too much sodium. The amount of sodium should not be more than double the calories.

Bean dips can be made quickly and easily in a blender or food processor. Experiment with different beans and different seasonings. Always drain and rinse the beans.

A dash of salt and 1½ tsp. of olive oil can be added to all these recipes to boost the flavor.

White Bean and Sun Dried Tomato Dip (M)

1 can (15 oz) cannellini or white beans

10 sun dried tomatoes, chopped

1 tsp. fresh rosemary

½ tsp. dried sage

1½ tsp. fresh lemon juice

1 clove garlic, minced

Add ingredients to a food processor or blender and blend until smooth.

White Bean and Roasted Pepper Dip (M)

1 can (15 oz) white beans

½ cup roasted bell peppers, fresh or jarred

1 clove garlic, minced

Add ingredients to a food processor or blender and blend until smooth.

Spicy Black Bean Dip (M)

1 can (15 oz) black beans

¾ tsp. cumin powder

½ tsp. coriander or 1 small bunch fresh cilantro

1 clove garlic, minced

3 tsp. fresh lemon juice

hot sauce to taste

Add ingredients to a food processor or blender and blend until smooth.

White Bean and Carrot Dip (P)

1 can (15 oz) white beans

1 cup carrots, mashed (steamed or roasted)

1 tsp. ground fennel seed or ground rosemary

Mix ingredients and serve.

White Bean "Tapenade" (M)

1 can (15 oz) white beans, blended

10 sun dried tomatoes, chopped

10 Kalamata olives, chopped or 1 Tbs. capers

Mix ingredients and serve.

Beanie Brownies (M)

Makes 12

For minty brownies, add ½ tsp. peppermint extract.

1 can (15 oz) black beans, drained and rinsed

2 Tbs. unsweetened cocoa powder, preferably alkaline free

½ cup quick oats

¼ tsp. sea salt

½ cup pure maple syrup

¼ cup coconut oil

2 tsp. pure vanilla extract

½ tsp. aluminum-free baking powder

½ cup cocoa nibs or chocolate chips
(if using chocolate chips be sure to use pure chips, no junk!)

½ – 1 cup walnuts or hazelnuts, chopped

Preheat oven to 350°. In food processor, combine all ingredients except chocolate nibs and nuts; blend until completely smooth. Stir in the nibs and ¾ of the nuts, then pour into a greased 8" × 8" pan. Top with remaining nuts. Cook 15 – 18 minutes.

Cool completely before cutting.

Meats

Meats

While on the program, meats will be poultry, buffalo, beef, white fish, and salmon. It is best if all fish is wild caught. Poultry, buffalo and beef should be free range and free of antibiotics, hormones etc. When eating an animal source we are also eating what that animal ate. So, for reference purposes a list of 'clean' and 'unclean' animals is included in this section. Clean animals are those feeding on vegetation. Unclean animals are bottom feeders of the sea or the yard keeper on land. When cows and chickens are fed hormones to make them fatter, we in turn ingest these hormones thus creating a variety of health issues. Pork is avoided because pigs cannot sweat and are therefore, unable to release toxins. They are also carriers of parasites that do not die even when the pork is cooked. Wild caught fish is important because farm raised fish are fed grains and additives. Quality meat and fish may cost a bit more but it's a wise investment in your health. There are a few selections in the Salads section which contain meat as does the Collard Green Minera in the Vegetables section. When cooking meats, adjust some of your own recipes by eliminating frying and substituting or omitting ingredients, such as BBQ sauces or spicy herbs.

Remember proper food combining; eat meats with vegetables and not starches. Keep total intake of animal protein (including cheese and eggs) to 12 – 14 oz per week. *The China Study* by Colin Campbell, PhD is a thorough resource regarding health and animal protein.

Unclean Meats

When it comes to sea creatures; bottom dwellers, such as lobsters and crabs, scavenge for dead animals on the sea floor. Shellfish such as oysters, clams and mussels similarly consume decaying organic matter that sinks to the sea floor, including sewage.

A common denominator of many of the animals designated as unclean is that they routinely eat flesh that would sicken or kill human beings. When we eat such animals we partake of a food chain that includes things harmful to people.

Many beef producers add growth hormones to cattle feed. Those hormones are passed along directly to the consumer's body. Some have even mingled manure and portions of unusable cattle carcass back into the feed to reduce costs and increase profits. These feeding practices can then make an otherwise clean classified animal now unclean and unsafe for human consumption. Imagine a cow chewing on itself or its own kind. Such detestable practices are generally considered to be the cause of Bovine Spongiform Encephalopathy, or BSE (mad cow's disease). Here are some references on the subject:

- Epidemiological studies conducted in the UK suggest that the source of BSE was cattle feed prepared from bovine tissues, such as brain and spinal cord, that was contaminated by the BSE agent. (Source: World Health Organization)
- We see a rising trend in unsafe meat production. Common sense dictates, to the best of our abilities, we should know the source and quality of the meat we eat. This includes fish and poultry. If chickens are raised in over-populated coops or fish drawn from mercury-polluted waters, they should not be eaten.
  (Source: www.planetpace.com)

Grilled Cilantro Chicken (P)

Saundra Lemaster

Serves 2

2 chicken breasts

1 large lime or 3 key limes per breast, enough to cover ¾ of chicken

1 bunch fresh cilantro, chopped

2 cloves garlic, minced

Serve with grilled vegetables and/or salad.

Lay one chicken breast at a time between two layers of plastic wrap or wax paper. Pound until breast is thin, being careful not to make holes through meat. In large covered container prepare marinade: lime juice, cilantro and garlic. In sealed plastic ware container, marinate chicken 2 – 3 hours; flip container and marinate another 2 – 3 hours. Heat grill on high. Sear both sides for 1 minute. Turn grill to medium. Cook approximately 3 minutes per side, basting with lemon and cilantro marinade. Citrus juices accelerate cooking. Take care not to over cook chicken.

Optional toppings:

- Fresh chopped cilantro
- Blend 1 avocado, 1 cup fresh cilantro, and water to desired consistency

Note: To keep animal protein reduced, cut breast into cutlets or purchase cutlets and do not pound.

Grilled Chicken with Gourmet Herb Sauce (P)

Serves 2

2 chicken cutlets (you can also cut 1 breast into 2 pieces)

1 cup plain goat yogurt

1 Tbs. fresh basil, finely chopped

½ heaping Tbs. dried parsley

½ heaping tsp. dried oregano

¼ heaping tsp. dried tarragon

1 tsp. fresh lemon juice

Mix last 6 ingredients for sauce. Refrigerate overnight to marry flavors. Bring to room temperature while preparing chicken. Preheat grill to medium. Grill chicken approximately 7 – 10 minutes per side until cooked thoroughly. When ready to serve, cut into slices. Smother with sauce.

Note: Substitute yogurt for 8 – 10 artichoke hearts (frozen or in jar) for proper food combining.

Spinach Stuffed Chicken Breast (P)

Serves 2

2 chicken breasts

3 cups fresh spinach, wilt in dry skillet

½ cup sheep or goat feta cheese (optional)

2 artichoke hearts, chopped,
(frozen and defrosted or jarred in water)

juice of ½ lemon

½ tsp. dried oregano

½ tsp. dried rosemary or fennel (optional)

Preheat oven 350°. Lay one chicken breast at a time between two layers of plastic wrap or wax paper. Pound breast thin, being careful not to make holes through the meat. Squeeze lemon juice over chicken, sprinkle with oregano. Let marinate while preparing stuffing or marinate for a couple hours.

In bowl, mix spinach, cheese, and artichoke hearts. Additional oregano and/or rosemary may be added. Separate mixture in half, squeeze out excess liquid with hands. Press mixture together. Put spinach mixture in center of each breast. Roll tightly, secure with toothpick or cooking band or press onto pan with seam side down. Bake approximately 20 minutes, depending on thickness of chicken breast.

Note: Omit cheese for proper food combining.

If staying with reduced animal protein, use 1 chicken breast for 2 people or eat ½ the breast and add chopped leftovers to salad for lunch.

Craig's Honduras Chicken Ⓜ

Serves 4 – 6

As a Peace Corps Volunteer, our son lived in the remote mountains of Honduras for a year before the US pulled out all volunteers due to escalated violence. Craig loves to cook and is blessed with creative culinary skills and enjoyed the culinary options in Washington, DC where he lived. But Honduras was no Washington, DC, nor were the food options. Here is a recipe he put together for the ever-abundant Honduran chicken.

- 1 whole, uncooked chicken (about 4 lbs)
- 2 in. fresh ginger (must be fresh)
- 5 cloves garlic (up to 10 if you want extra garlic)
- ½ cup honey
- ¼ cup inexpensive white wine or sherry

Rinse chicken, including the inside. Put in pot large enough to fit with a tight lid. Combine remaining ingredients in small bowl for marinade. Rub marinade under chicken skin, making sure to get tiny pieces of garlic and ginger in there too. Baste the outside of chicken with remaining juices. I recommend doing this inside the pot because all the marinade needs to make its way into the pot.

There must be a small puddle of liquid or your chicken will burn and you will ruin your pot. If there isn't enough liquid, add more wine/sherry or water. Add more honey for sweeter preferences. Fats from chicken will join the liquid and prevent sticking.

Cook on low for about an hour up to an hour and a half. The liquid will reduce into a delicious sweet sauce and caramelize in the process. It can be spooned on top of chicken when serving.

Serve with salad or vegetables.

Ukrainian Chicken (P)

Serves 4-6

1 whole chicken

1 bay leaf

Especially good with Master Veggie Mix I and II Salads.

Place chicken and bay leaf in roaster pan. Roast in tightly-sealed pan on low heat or in an oven at 325°. For chicken under 4 lbs, cook approximately 1 ½ hours; if over 4 lbs, cook 1 ¾ hours.

When cool enough to handle, remove chicken from pan. Drain juices into a large mug.

Refrigerate until fat congeals on top then remove congealed fat and discard. Meanwhile, remove meat from the chicken and cut into bite-size pieces. Reheat jelled broth.

Remove bay leaf and pour juices over cut up chicken; completely covering chicken. Depending on the amount of broth, only half the chicken might be used. Refrigerate until chicken and juice are jelled, serve cold.

Note: Chicken may also be cooked whole in a crock pot. This takes approximately 4 hours.

Easy Crock pot Chicken or Turkey (P)

Serves 6

3 chicken or turkey breasts, skinless

3 cloves garlic, chopped

½ red onion, diced

2 celery stalks, trimmed, chopped

4 small carrots, sliced

2 fennel bulbs, trimmed, cubed
or 2 kohlrabi, peeled, cubed

Italian style herbs, to taste
(basil, rosemary, thyme, marjoram)

fresh filtered water, as needed

fresh parsley, chopped, for garnish

Turn crock pot on high. Rinse chicken or turkey breast in cold water, remove skin. Place in bottom of crock pot. Top with remaining ingredients. Pour filtered water over poultry and vegetables until completely submerged. Cover. Cook on high 4 – 5 hours or until the meat falls apart when tested with a fork.

Pull cooked poultry apart into strings or serve whole. Serve with a sprinkling of fresh chopped parsley.

Turkey Meatloaf (P)

Serves 4 – 6

For extra flavor, use only arugula instead of spinach.

1 lb ground turkey
(dark meat is preferable)

10 oz. container fresh spinach
(or half spinach, half arugula), wilted

sheep feta, about ½ cup

dried oregano

dried parsley

½ medium onion, chopped

1 cup shredded vegetables such as carrots, zucchini, celery

1 tsp. whole fennel seed

8 – 10 cloves garlic, minced

fresh ground black pepper

Sprinkle one side of the feta heavily with oregano and the other with parsley. Press into cheese. Note: If you can't find the feta in slabs then add the oregano, parsley, and cheese directly to the meat mixture. Cut cheese into cubes and spread onto a shallow pan with sides. Bake at 350° about 10 minutes. The cheese will not melt but will get very soft. Remove from oven and prop a towel under one side so water drains from cheese. Let cool. Wilt spinach on low without oil, or use ½ spinach and ½ arugula. When wilted, set aside to cool.

Mix mix all ingredients with turkey including sautéed onion and shredded vegetables. Put in single loaf pan, shape a rectangle by hand on baking sheet, or press into muffin tins. If using a single loaf pan, bake at 350° for about 45 minutes (less time for the smaller pans). For added flavor and/or presentation, wrap loaf with turkey bacon and secure with toothpicks or carrot sticks before baking.

Note: Omit cheese for proper food combining.

Kabobs Ⓟ

Serves 2

wooden or metal skewers

1 large chicken breast or equivalent beef portion

vegetables of choice
(review Vegetable Kabobs in Vegetables section)

juice of 1 fresh lemon

½ tsp. ground rosemary or oregano

3 cloves garlic, minced

Combine lemon juice, garlic and herbs to make marinade. Cut breast into 1 inch chunks and marinate 1 – 2 hours. If using beef, do not marinate but press minced garlic and/or spices into meat. Lightly oil cut vegetables and sprinkle with spices of choice. Preheat grill to medium. Alternately skewer meat and vegetables. Grill approximately 5 minutes per side or until meat in cooked. Serve alone or on a bed of greens.

Stuffed Cabbage Leaves (P)

Makes approximately 25 – 30 rolls

1 large, green cabbage or collard greens

1 lb. cooked ground beef, shredded chicken, or ground turkey

10 oz. fresh spinach, sautéed, or frozen and defrosted (squeeze out liquid)

1 Tbs. fresh mint, finely chopped

6 cloves garlic, minced

1 cup zucchini, finely chopped

½ cup fresh parsley, finely chopped

1 Tbs. dried fennel seed

filtered water

juice of 1 lemon (about 4 Tbs.)

Cut out core of cabbage. Stick a large fork into center. Bring large pot of filtered water to a boil. Immerse cabbage, leaving fork in place. When outer leaves turn bright green, remove from pan. Using fork, gently peel away softened leaves. Return to pot. Repeat until all cabbage leaves have been removed.

If using collared greens, blanch leaves in hot water until softened and darker green. Gently shave down thick stems if desired. Cut very large leaves in half.

Mix all ingredients. Set aside.

To make rolls, fill leaf with heaping tablespoon of stuffing. Place stuffing 1 inch from thick end of cabbage leaf. Fold bottom over filling, fold sides in, roll up. For smaller rolls, fill with heaping teaspoon of stuffing.

(Recipe continues on next page.)

Preheat oven to 350°. In large baking dish, place rolls closely together, seam side down. Layer if necessary. Add lemon juice to enough water to cover bottom of dish. Baste a few times during cooking. Bake uncovered 30 – 45 minutes. May also be eaten at room temperature.

Variation for extra flavor:
- *Use Artichoke Sauce recipe in Dressings section as a topping when serving*
- *Add feta cheese to filling mix*

Grilled Salmon and Zucchini (P)

Serves 2

2 salmon steaks, about ¼ lb. each

2 medium zucchini, sliced

4 Tbs. lemon juice

½ tsp. garlic powder

1 tsp. dill weed

Make a marinade of oil, lemon juice, and seasonings and marinate the salmon steaks for half an hour, turning once or twice. Place both salmon and zucchini on grill (or under broiler) and cook salmon for about 4 minutes on each side. Baste both salmon and zucchini with marinade. Cook until just done.

Note: Grouper and tuna are good substitutes for the salmon.

Wild caught Alaskan salmon is the way to go. Avoid farm-raised fish. Salmon is high in Omega-3 and has DHA and EPA. Avocados are high in Vitamin E and glutathione. Eating salmon also increases the absorption of carotenoids and lowers cholesterol. Bon appétit!

Grilled Salmon with Avocado Dip (M)

Serves 4

1 ripe avocado, peeled, pitted and diced

2 cloves garlic, peeled and minced

3 Tbs. plain goat yogurt

1 Tbs. fresh lemon juice

1 lb wild caught salmon steaks

2 tsp. dried dill weed

1 tsp. lemon zest

Preheat an outdoor grill on high heat. Lightly oil grate.

In a medium bowl, mash together avocados, garlic, yogurt, and lemon juice. Season with salt and pepper.

Rub salmon with dill and lemon zest. Place salmon skin side up on prepared grill. Cook approximately 15 minutes. Turn, and grill until easily flaked with a fork. Serve with Avocado Dip.

Note: For proper food combining, omit goat yogurt and avocado.

Grilled Yellow Fin Tuna (P)

Serves 4

1 lb fresh or frozen, wild caught tuna steaks, boneless/skinless

extra-virgin olive oil

fresh lime or lemon

English cucumber, thinly sliced

fresh dill

Mix cucumber, dill, and lime or lemon juice; set aside.

Dry steaks with paper towels, rub with olive oil. Preheat grill on high. With long tongs, place tuna steaks on grill. Do *not* disturb for at least 2 – 3 minutes. Turn steaks 45 degrees (quarter turn), leave them for another 2 minutes. (This is to give steaks that pretty diamond pattern seen in fancy restaurants.) Turn steaks over. Grill for another 3 – 4 minutes. Do not overcook tuna; it will become dry. Drizzle with lemon or lime juice.

Top with cucumber mixture and serve.

Baked Fish Florentine Ⓟ

Serves 4

1 small onion, thinly sliced

4 cloves garlic, chopped

1 package frozen artichoke hearts, thawed and drained or 1 jar in water, about 9 oz

1 tsp. organic lemon zest

⅔ cup low sodium vegetable broth or water

juice of one lemon

4 small fillets (4 oz. each) of white fish or wild salmon

20 oz. baby spinach

Preheat oven to 425°. Sauté onion and garlic on low/medium so they cook in their own juices until soft, add water if necessary to keep from sticking. Add artichoke hearts, lemon zest, lemon juice and vegetable broth. Simmer uncovered over medium/high heat, stirring occasionally, reducing sauce. Rinse fish and pat dry. Transfer mixture to a baking dish. Arrange fish over the mixture in single layer. Cover dish tightly with foil. Bake about 12 – 15 minutes.

While fish is baking, sauté spinach in pan on low so it cooks in its own juices or add a touch of lemon or water if it sticks. Cook until wilted. Serve fish on top of spinach bed.

The ingredients can also be cooked all together. Layer raw spinach in a baking dish and top with fish. In a bowl, mix onion, garlic, artichokes, zest, and lemon juice. There is no need for the broth. Pour mixture over the fish and bake as directed above.

Salads

Salads

The options are limitless! Think outside the box; think about warm salads, pasta salads, hot grains mixed with cold greens, shredded vegetable salads. Forget about the old salads of lettuce, tomato and cucumber with Ranch dressing! You are on to new salad horizons! You are not limited to what is considered usual. There are many recipes that don't even contain greens. Think non-traditional; it will enhance your salad repertoire considerably and excite your taste buds.

Greens are still the most nutritious food choice for health and weight loss. Per calorie there is more calcium and protein in some vegetables then milk or beef. Because of their low caloric count you do not have to limit portions, count calories, or weigh food. Salads are rapidly digested due to their high water content and live enzymes. There are mixed philosophies regarding when to eat a salad and how much raw food is best. Some believe it is best to eat a salad after a meal because the live enzymes will help digest the cooked food. Enzymes are still living in raw foods and contain more nutrients than their cooked counterparts. For those with healthier digestive tracts, maintaining a lifestyle of 75% – 80% raw is a healthful choice. However, depending on digestive issues, a predominantly cooked diet is best until healing takes place.

Salad are versatile, easy, nutritious and yummy! So get yourself some greens, experiment, and have fun.

Salad Tips

- Substitute or add other greens for romaine, Bibb, baby spinach, mixed greens, arugula or kale.
- Combine whatever you have on hand, such as frozen peas, hearts of palm, black olives, avocado and cucumbers with lemon juice… so yummy.
- For something heartier, add rice or beans.
- Turn leftovers, like chili, into an entrée by putting it on top of a bed of greens.
- Avoid store bought dressing; use dressing recipes in the Dressings/Sauce/Dip section. You will be surprised when you no longer like a bottled dressing. Lemon juice, Braggs, garlic and olive oil make a great dressing. The easiest is still fresh squeezed lemon juice. Raw nuts and fruit are a fast and easy dressing.
- Boxed greens are always convenient, but if time is not a constraint, then prep and store lettuce in advance. Romaine lettuce and other greens can be washed and patted dry or spun dry then stored in zip-lock bags or plastic ware. Inserting a paper towel (dry) helps keep greens fresh for several days.
- Save time throughout the week by shopping and prepping on the same day. Feel free to cheat and use a food processor! Simply chop various vegetables (such as the Veggie Mix salads in this chapter) and store them separately in jars in the fridge. It's a great idea shared by my friend JoAnn Lowell. This allows you to grab a variety of vegetables to whip up a salad, cook a side of vegetables or make a fast soup.

English Cucumber (P)

Serves 1

1 English cucumber, diced

4 artichoke hearts, chopped, frozen and defrosted or jarred in water

3 – 4 celery stalks, diced

fresh lime juice, to taste

drizzle of olive oil

sheep or goat cheese, crumbled

Black or Kalamata olives (optional)

¼ cup frozen peas, defrosted (optional)

Mix all ingredients in bowl. Toss lightly and serve.

Greek Cucumber (P)

Serves 3-4

> *A fantastic treat is to broil the cheese first.*

1 large English cucumber, diced

¼ cup fresh dill, chopped

½ tsp. dried oregano

¼ – ⅓ cup crumbled goat or sheep feta

1 Tbs. olive oil

Combine cucumber, dill and oregano in bowl. Toss. Add oil and lemon juice in small bowl, mix with cucumber mixture. Add cheese, gently toss again.

A fantastic treat is to broil the cheese first. If you can find authentic goat or sheep feta in a slab, coat each side with dried oregano and gently push the oregano into the cheese using your fingertips. Broil on medium/high. Watch it closely so it doesn't burn. Let it cool; it will become much firmer. Drain off any water that is formed. Toss into salad.

Tzatziki Yogurt Cucumber Salad (P)

Serves 1

½ cup plain goat yogurt, strained

1 cucumber, English cucumber preferred
(if using regular cucumber, remove seeds as it can be too watery)

½ clove garlic, finely minced

1 – 2 Tbs. fresh mint, roughly chopped

3 Tbs. fresh dill, both stems and fronds, chopped (or to taste)

juice of half a lemon, about 1 ½ Tbs.

Strain yogurt through a fine sieve or through a coffee filter in a colander suspended over a bowl. It will take an hour or so. If you want even creamier yogurt (your personal preference), drain until it stops dripping. Peel cucumbers and remove seeds (unless English cucumber is used). Coarsely grate on standard kitchen box grater. Combine all ingredients. Best if refrigerated to allow flavors to marry, but can also be used as a last-minute side or dip.

Avocado Pesto Stuffed Cucumber (P)

Serves 2

1 English cucumber

3 cloves garlic, minced

1 Tbs. pine nuts

1 tsp. fresh lemon juice

15 large fresh basil leaves, chopped fine

1 avocado, scoop out flesh

Cut cucumber in half lengthwise, with melon baller or spoon, scoop out seeds, discard. Continue scooping cucumber to leave ¼ inch shell. In blender add removed pieces of cucumber, garlic, basil, pine nuts. Add lemon juice. Blend until smooth. Fork mash avocado. Add avocado to mixture. Mix well. Fill cucumber channels evenly. Garnish with chopped basil.

Note: Pine nuts do not technically combine properly with avocado.

Cuc-Zuc (P)

Serves 1

½ English cucumber, chopped
6 Kalamata olives, pitted
½ zucchini, chopped or shredded
¼ cup sheep or goat cheese, crumbled
lime juice to taste
drizzle of olive oil
⅛ cup fresh basil, chopped

Put first 3 ingredients in bowl. Toss with fresh lime juice and olive oil. Top with cheese and basil. Serve immediately.

Variations
- *Serve on bed of greens: baby spinach, arugula, baby greens, watercress or mixed greens.*
- *Add thinly sliced beef or chicken.*
- *Add other vegetables of choice.*

Pea-Cumber (P)

Serves 4

16 oz. package frozen peas, thawed

15 oz. jar artichoke hearts, water packed or 8 frozen, defrosted artichoke hearts, chopped

1 English cucumber, diced

juice one fresh lemon, to taste

drizzle of olive oil

Mix all ingredients in bowl. Toss if eating immediately. If making for later, store in refrigerator without adding lemon juice. Lemon juice looses its flavor during refrigeration. So it is always best to dress a salad immediately prior to eating.

Variations

- *Add chopped parsley, cilantro and/or dill*
- *Omit artichoke hearts*
- *Add sliced black olives with or without artichoke hearts*
- *Add shredded carrot*
- *Add 2 Tablespoons each mint and basil*

Crispy Sugar Snap Pea Salad (P)

Serves 4

> *Snap peas may also be used raw instead of steamed.*

½ lb sugar snap peas, trimmed

1 English cucumber, halved lengthwise

1 lb red radishes (or substitute daikon)

¼ cup sesame seeds, raw or toasted (optional)

1 Tbs. fresh lemon or lime juice

Herb of choice – fresh , recommended

Wash and snap off the stem end of each pea pod, pulling down the length of the pod to remove the string (some varieties have strings on both sides). Steam about 30 seconds, or just until they turn bright green. Plunge into cold water to stop cooking. Drain. Cut cucumber and radishes crosswise into ¼ inch thick slices. Toss with remaining ingredients and serve.

Kale Salad (M)

Serves 3

4 cups raw kale, thinly sliced without stem

2 cups raw cabbage, shredded

1 cup raw carrot, shredded

2 – 4 Tbs. vinegar, raw apple cider

2 – 4 Tbs. Braggs

2 Tbs. extra virgin olive oil

"Massaging" the vegetables is key to softening them up.

Mix the first 3 ingredients. Amounts are approximate in amount and according to personal preference. Add last 3 ingredients by hand, rubbing between finger tips. For the seasoning amounts, start with 2 Tbs. and go up from there as you taste. Remember the taste will intensify a bit as it sits. Chill for 1 hour to let vegetables soften.

Raw Asparagus & Kale "Guacamole" Salad Ⓟ

Serves 2

1 large ripe avocado

1 Tbs. fresh-squeezed lemon juice

pinch sea salt

6 asparagus spears, chopped

3 – 4 kale leaves, sliced – dinosaur kale preferred

1 celery stalk, thinly sliced

1 green onion, diced

¼ cup raw pumpkin seeds

fresh cilantro leaves

Wash avocado, kale, asparagus and celery. Mash together avocado, lemon juice and sea salt in a bowl. Remove woody ends from bottom of asparagus spears and thinly slice diagonally (¼ inch). Tips may be chopped or left whole to be used as a garnish. Cut kale in ½ inch strips across the vein. Thinly slice celery. Combine all ingredients, adding cilantro to taste.

Note: Pumpkin seeds technically do not combine properly with avocado.

Stuffed Avocado (P)

Serves 2

For extra flavor, add chopped artichoke hearts or black olives.

1 Hass avocado

¼ English cucumber, chopped

1 tsp. ground rosemary or
1 Tbs. fresh chopped basil or cilantro

2 Tbs. fresh lemon or lime juice

Mix lemon/lime juice with rosemary to let flavors marry while preparing avocado.

Slice avocado around the center lengthwise, twist to separate the halves. Holding one half in the palm of your hand or lay it on a cutting board. With a sharp, straight edge knife hit the pit so the knife lodges in the pit. Twist knife to remove nut. Score the avocado, being careful not to pierce the skin. Using a spoon, carefully scoop out the avocado, leaving the skin intact.

Add all ingredients in a bowl and toss gently. Refill avocado skins with mixture. Garnish with chopped herbs.

Sweet Slaw (P)

Serves 6 – 8

1 small green cabbage, shredded

3 – 4 carrots, grated

2 crunchy, sweet apples, cored, chopped

1 cup walnuts, chopped

These amounts are estimates; adjust according to personal taste. Mix all ingredients in large bowl. Store tightly covered in refrigerator without dressing of any kind. Slaw will stay fresh 3 – 4 days. Use as needed, mixing with options from the Dressings, Sauces & Dips section.

Grated Carrot (P)

Serves 1

1 raw carrot, unpeeled, washed, finely grated

1 tsp. lemon juice, to taste

½ – 1 tsp. approved sweetener

1 – 2 Tbs. nuts, chopped (optional)

Combine lime juice and sweetener to taste. Add grated carrot. Toss. Serve immediately.

Note: It makes a world of difference if the carrot in finely grated, as opposed to being medium or coarsely grated.

Beet Salad (P)

Serves 2

1 lb beets

¼ cup of fresh lemon juice

1 clove garlic, finely minced

1 – 2 Tbs. onion, finely minced

1 tsp. extra virgin olive oil, (optional)

¼ cup crumbled sheep or goat feta (optional)

There are different ways to cook beets. Peel, cube and steam beets. Or leave unpeeled and steam whole or cut. If you leave the peel on: after they are cooked, run them under tepid water and rub the peel off with your finger tips, cube. Marinate cubed beets in lemon juice, for a few hours or overnight. When ready to serve mix minced garlic and minced onion in a bowl with olive oil and pour it over the beets on the plate. Just put the onion and garlic on top of the beets when you are ready to serve; do not mix it all or the onions and garlic will turn red. Serve cold or at room temperature.

Variation

Peel an orange down to the meat, remove all membranes, and slice. Arrange beets on plate then place oranges on top.

Broccoli Apple Salad (P)

Serves 3

1 apple, cored, chopped

¼ cup walnuts, chopped

1 ½ cups frozen broccoli, defrosted, chopped

dressing (from Dressings, Sauces & Dips section)

Mix all ingredients in bowl. Toss with dressing of choice. Creamy Apple Almond Dressing is great with this salad.

Note: Using frozen broccoli allows for salad prepared in the morning to be defrosted and ready to be dressed by lunch time.

Spinach and Asian Pear Salad (P)

Serves 2

⅔ cups walnuts or pecans, chopped

1 ½ Tbs. fresh lemon juice

¼ tsp. acceptable sweetener

3 cups fresh baby spinach

1 Asian pear, cored and sliced thin

Asian pears originated and have been grown in Asia for at least 3,000 years. They are sweet with low acid, crisp, and have a juicy texture.

Combine ⅓ cup nuts in blender with lemon juice and sweetener, blend until smooth. Mix spinach, remaining nuts, and pear slices in bowl, add dressing. Toss to coat.

Hijiki Seaweed Rollup Ⓟ

Serves 4

> *Most seaweed is high in essential amino acids, which makes it a valuable source of vegetable protein. Seaweeds contain vitamins A, C & B-12, potassium, iron, calcium, iodine, and magnesium.*

1 nori sheet per person (dried seaweed for rolling)

1 cup cooked brown rice

2 ½ Tbs. dried Hijiki (substitute other seaweed if desired)

1 lb frozen edamame, defrosted (non GMO only)

1 Tbs. olive oil

1 tsp. sesame oil (not toasted)

⅛ cup fresh lemon juice

1 Tbs. accepted sweetener

½ daikon radish, about the size of a large carrot, peeled, shredded

1 large carrot, shredded

4 handfuls baby spinach

Rehydrate Hijiki in a bowl of hot water for approximately 20 minutes. It will double in volume so use a bowl that is big enough. To make dressing, mix both oils, sweetener, lemon juice. Set aside. Use vegetable peeler to peel carrot and daikon into strips or cut into matchsticks. In large bowl, toss greens, Hijiki, carrot, daikon and edamame. Add dressing slowly, just enough to lightly coat vegetables. Add hot rice.

Put mixture across one end of the nori sheet, roll tightly. Moisten your finger tip with water to moisten the finished end, it will stick to itself. Eat like a burrito or using a very sharp knife, cut into rolls like sushi. Vegetables can also be rolled alone by omitting rice.

Note: If you prefer not to have hot mixed with cold, cook rice ahead and refrigerate prior to making.

Watercress (P)

Serves 2

1 bunch hydroponic watercress, cut with scissors

1 small English cucumber, diced

8 Kalamata olives, sliced

goat or sheep feta cheese

extra virgin olive oil

fresh lemon juice

Hydroponic watercress is preferable because of freshness. If unavailable, use watercress that is not wilted in any way.

Mix first 3 ingredients in large bowl. Vary amount of olives according to personal taste. Drizzle ingredients lightly with olive oil, a squeeze of lemon. Toss well. Add feta cheese last. Toss again.

Squash-n-Hearts (P)

Serves 2

1 cup frozen peas, defrosted

3 artichoke hearts, chopped, frozen and defrosted or jarred in water

½ medium, yellow summer squash, shredded

2 cups fresh spinach, torn into bite size pieces

⅛ cup fresh parsley, chopped

3 – 4 Tbs. fresh lemon or lime juice

1 – 2 Tbs. olive oil

Spices or herbs of choice (optional)

Toss all ingredients in bowl, adjusting juice and olive oil according to personal taste.

Hearts of Palm (P)

Serves 3 – 4

To really amp up this salad, add chopped chicken.

1 jar hearts of palm, in water, sliced

2 celery stalks, diced

1 cup black olives, sliced

1 cup cucumber, diced

fresh lemon, to taste

Mix all ingredients in bowl.

Speared Hearts (P)

Serves 3 – 4

1 small bunch asparagus, about ¾ pound

one 14 ounce can or jar hearts of palm, in water, drained, sliced

⅓ cup black olives, sliced

1 Tbs. olive oil

1 Tbs. fresh lemon juice

½ tsp. dried tarragon or oregano

Mix oil, juice and spice. Set aside while preparing salad so the flavors marry. Wash asparagus, cut off tough ends. Grill, roast (directions for both can be found in Vegetables section) or blanch asparagus. Asparagus can be mixed while hot or cold. Mix all ingredients. Toss with oil mixture. Can be served topping a bed of greens, watercress, hot or cold rice.

Veggie Wraps (P)

1 – 2 rolls per serving

Optional fillings:

raw nut butters

shredded carrots

thin cucumber spears

thin zucchini or yellow squash spears

steamed asparagus

chopped apples or pears

slice of turkey or chicken

Use large romaine lettuce or other large leafy lettuce. Break off stem. Stack 2 leaves on top of each other with ends laying in opposite directions. Put a row of any of the optional fillings down the center and roll. Depending on the type of lettuce, it is easier to roll from side to side rather than from stem to top.

Experiment with raw (great crunch!) or slightly steamed collard greens.

Veggie Master Mixes (P)

Serves 2

> *Make a large batch to steam and use as a side vegetable.*

Veggie Master Mix I

- ½ cup frozen peas, thawed
- ½ cup frozen green beans, thawed
- ½ cup raw carrot, coarsely grated or sliced
- ½ cup broccoli florets
- ¼ cup broccoli stalk, coarsely shredded or sliced
- ¾ cup zucchini and/or yellow squash, diced or coarsely shredded
- 2 Tbs. red cabbage (for color), shredded
- ¾ cup green cabbage, shredded

Veggie Master Mix II

- ½ cup frozen peas, thawed
- ½ cup frozen green beans, thawed
- 1 cup zucchini, coarsely shredded
- 1 cup celery, chopped or sliced
- 1 cup green cabbage, shredded
- ½ English cucumber, diced

Optional Ingredients

- sugar snap peas, raw or lightly steamed
- 2 – 3 water packed artichoke hearts or frozen and defrosted, cut in halves or quarters
- ½ avocado, in large chunks
- apple, peach or pear, diced

(Recipe continues on next page)

Ingredient amounts are approximate. Add more or less of each ingredient according to your personal preference. Salad will keep for several days, if sealed tightly and refrigerated without added oil or other liquid.

Master Mixes can be eaten...

- as salad with or without added greens
- using fresh lime juice with a small amount extra-virgin olive oil for dressing
- lightly steamed, served as a side dish
- added to cooked rice, warmed through
- as soup, by adding to heated broth
- as filling for lettuce wraps
- with added grilled chicken, turkey, salmon or tuna

Crunchy Salad (P)

Serves 4

2 English cucumbers, cubed

4 large celery stalks, cubed

1 can (3.5 oz) black olives, sliced

1 jar artichoke hearts, in water not oil, quartered and chopped

5 Tbs. fresh mint, finely chopped

4 Tbs. fresh parsley, finely chopped

6 Tbs. fresh lime juice

sheep feta cheese (optional)

½ tsp. dried oregano

If you find the cheese in a slab form, completely cover both sides with oregano and gently press into cheese. Broil for 5 – 7 minutes, drain liquid and let cool.

Mix lime and ½ teaspoon oregano. Let liquids stand while preparing the salad. Mix all vegetables and herbs. Toss with dressing.

Grilled Romaine (P)

Serves 2

1 large head romaine lettuce

olive oil

spices of choice

lemon juice to garnish (optional)

Grill or broil lettuce, place 2 wedges on each plate. Top with salad fixings.

To prepare: Quarter the head of lettuce to end up with 4 long wedges. Slightly spritz or brush on olive oil so it gets in between the layers. Sprinkle with spices of choice.

To grill: preheat grill to medium/high. Grill cut side down for approximately 3-4 minutes. Be careful not to burn it but the edges should be browned. Place in serving plate, cut side up. Top with fixings.

To broil: follow "to prepare" directions as above. Place on cookie sheet. Broil on medium/high, cut side up until browned around edges. Follow serving suggestions as above.

Grilled or broiled romaine makes a unique foundation for a yummy salad. It can be eaten as a side vegetable as well.

When using grilled romaine as a salad base, choose any ingredients that you like for a salad and cut them ahead of time. Then simply use them to top the lettuce.

Chicken Salad (P)

Serves 1

> *Variation: Mix cilantro, lime, chicken and 1 mashed avocado. Then top greens.*

½ cup cooked chicken, chopped

2 cups romaine chopped,

½ cup cucumber, diced

1 small carrot, shredded

1 Tbs. fresh cilantro, chopped

2 artichoke hearts, chopped (frozen and defrosted or jarred in water)

Fresh lime, to taste, approximately 1 Tbs.

Mix vegetables and chicken in bowl. Squeeze lime. Toss and serve. Vary amounts depending on personal preference.

Herbed Chicken Salad

Serves 1

> *Don't skip this recipe if you don't have all the herbs. You can substitute with dill or basil. Find the blend you like best.*

½ cup cooked chicken, pulled or chopped

½ English cucumber, with peel, chopped

1 head of soft lettuce, like Boston lettuce, torn into bite size pieces

1 Tbs. each parsley, tarragon, chervil, chives and mint (fresh, not dried)

1 ½ – 2 Tbs. fresh lemon juice

Use left over chicken or bake 1 large chicken breast. In medium bowl mix lettuce, cucumber, herbs, toss with oil and juice to taste. Divide into serving plates, top with hot or cold chicken.

Steak Salad (P)

Serves 4

3 cups cooked string beans, see below*

10 oz. steak of choice, cooked, sliced thin

1 small onion, sliced thin

4 cups romaine or other lettuce, chopped

2 cups baby spinach

1 carrot, shredded

1 tsp. garlic, minced

½ tsp. dried thyme

½ tsp. salt free seasoning

1 Tbs. fresh lemon juice

fresh squeezed lemon

*Sauté fresh or frozen string beans on medium/low with garlic, thyme, salt free seasoning, one tablespoon fresh lemon juice and a little water to prevent sticking.

While cooking string beans, grill or broil steak. Cut into very thin diagonal strips, set aside, keeping warm. If using onion, slice, sauté on medium/low or slice to use raw.

Mix greens, carrots and onions (if using raw). Toss with fresh squeezed lemon to taste. Place greens on dinner plate. Top with hot green beans, steak and onions. Serve immediately.

Soups

Soups

Soups can be fun and easy or totally frustrating. The fun and easy part is just putting leftover meals in a pot of broth and having a new dinner ! Green Rice, Sweet Slaw, Asian Grain or Veggie Master Mix salads can all be made into soup by adding broth. The frustrating part can be making soup from scratch and getting the spices just right so there is no need for too much salt. It's easy to change flavor intensity and texture, thus actually creating a completely different soup. A standard broth soup can be turned into a creamy soup by pureeing the contents. Mix it up, puree all the contents or just half, depending on desired consistency. Even soups with meats can be pureed. Always cook soups on medium or medium/low. Boiling will destroy the nutritional content and enzymes. Avoid store bought soups; healthful options are not readily available. Most store bought soups are too high in sodium and fat. They are stored for too long and over cooked, reducing the nutritional value. Make a large pot of broth and freeze it in serving sizes you would normally use for soup. Freezer bags work great for freezing broth and soups. Of course your freezer is neater if you use plastic containers and stack them. Never put hot liquid into a plastic container; wait until it is completely cooled. Making a big pot of soup and freezing it is also a great way to make sure you utilize your cooking time to its maximum potential. Freezing soups will always provide an instant lunch or supper. If using store bought broth is necessary, keep the sodium to 300 mg per serving.

Dairy-free Cream Soups

Personally, I prefer the texture of cream soups over broth soups. Without being able to have dairy, options were once limited. But cauliflower has saved the cream soup day! Besides the fact that it is a cruciferous vegetable and very nutritious, it lends itself nicely to a creamy appearance and texture. Cauliflower can be pureed in water, nut milks, or broths for a soup base.

The soup recipes that feature cauliflower are illustrations of how you can personalize any dish with a few simple changes. For example, the Fish Chowder is wonderful, but if you aren't a fish eater, don't despair; it tastes fantastic without the fish! You can also experiment by substituting carrots for cauliflower to have a creamy carrot base for soup.

In order to combine properly, do not add fish or meat to an almond milk base, but rather use chicken or vegetable broth.

Cauliflower Soup Base (P)

Serves 2

1 cauliflower head, chopped

2 cups almond milk

1 clove garlic

¼ cup cashews (optional)

Tarragon lends a sweet taste, especially if not using almond milk. Fennel or cardamom add a fun twist.

This soup can be eaten this way or use it as a base to build from. Here are some tips: cook and puree other vegetables with the cauliflower, reserve some of the cooked vegetables and add them back into the pureed soup, increase liquid and add baby spinach at the end until it wilts, use whatever herbs/spices you prefer, or add turkey bacon or sausage.

Add all ingredients except nuts/seeds to pot and cook on low, until cauliflower is tender.

In increments, puree soup in food processor or blender. Be very careful about the steam, it can blow the cover off the blender! Blend the nuts and some of the almond milk in the blender separately to insure all the nuts are blended smooth. Add to soup. For presentation; top soup with finely chopped nuts.

Creamy Cauliflower Soup (P)

Serves 2

1 cauliflower head, cut into 1 inch pieces;
set ¼ of the cauliflower aside

2 cups water or broth or almond milk

3 carrots, cut into 1 inch pieces

3 carrots, cut into very thin circles, about ⅛ in.

olive oil

spice of choice (optional)

In a bowl, place ¼ of the cut cauliflower and the carrots cut into circles. Coat hands with olive oil and rub vegetables. Spread out onto a cookie sheet; do not layer them. Roast in a preheated oven at 450° until tender when pierced with a fork. Put aside.

While vegetables are roasting, put the remainder of cauliflower, remainder of carrots, liquid and any spices or herbs into a stock pan and simmer until vegetables are completely soft. In increments, puree soup in food processor or blender. Be very careful about the steam, it will blow the cover off the blender! Add roasted vegetables to pureed soup. Serve.

Variations

- *Add frozen peas into soup when adding roasted vegetables*
- *Omit the carrots and add peas at the end*

Vegetable Broth (P)

Makes about 6 cups

2 medium carrots

1 medium parsnip

1 cup celeriac (celery root), peeled or 1 small head celery

3 cloves garlic, unpeeled, minced

½ cup fresh parsley

2 bay leaves

4 fresh sprigs rosemary

6 fresh sprigs oregano

½ tsp. black pepper

8 cups filtered water

Wash all vegetables well but do not peel, except peel celeriac. Coarsely chop all vegetables. Add vegetables to water in stock pan. Bring to a boil. Reduce heat to medium, simmering until all vegetables are tender. Add spices and herbs, including stems. Continue to simmer, covered on low for 1 hour.

Strain stock though fine mesh colander into large pan or bowl. Press cooked vegetables through with the back of a large, serving spoon to release liquids remaining in vegetables.

Broth will keep refrigerated 3 days. Broth can be frozen in large freezer bags. Label bags with quantity amount.

Speedy Vegetable Soup (P)

Serves 4

32 oz. organic, low sodium chicken
or vegetable broth

1 cup frozen peas

1 cup frozen broccoli

1 cup frozen spinach

drizzle fresh lemon juice (optional)

herbs of choice – basil, oregano, fennel, parsley, tarragon

Place all ingredients in pan and heat until hot. Serve. Drizzle lemon for a little twist. Enjoy!

Hearty Vegetable Soup (P)

Serves 4

If desired, garnish with finely grated carrot.

32 oz. chicken broth

½ cup broccoli stems,
coarsely shredded

½ cup broccoli florets, chopped

2 cups green cabbage, thinly sliced

½ cup fresh or frozen green beans, 1 inch pieces

1 cup zucchini (or mix of zucchini and yellow squash), chopped

1 large handful raw baby spinach

Cook broccoli stems in broth until al dente. Add remaining vegetables except spinach. Cook until vegetables are tender, approximately 10 minutes. Add spinach. Turn heat off; allow spinach to wilt. Ladle into bowls.

Roasted Vegetable Soup (P)

Serves 4

32 oz. organic, low sodium chicken broth

4 cups roasted vegetables

spices/herbs of choice

Follow recipe for roasting vegetables in Vegetables section. Puree half the vegetables. Add puree and remaining roasted vegetables to broth. Add more spices/herbs (in addition to the spices/herbs on roasted vegetables) to soup. Heat. To thicken soup, puree additional vegetables.

Vegetables to roast alone or in any combination:

- *asparagus and string beans*
- *broccoli and cauliflower*
- *carrot and fennel*
- *zucchini, summer squash, and butternut squash*
- *garlic*

Vegetable Brown Rice Soup (P)

Recipe by Glenda Reece

Serves 6 – 8

45 oz. vegetable or chicken broth

½ cup cooked brown rice

2 – 3 cups frozen green beans

¾ head green cabbage, chopped or shredded

2 small carrots, chopped small

spices/herbs of choice

Place vegetables and stock in large stock pan. Cook on medium until vegetables are tender, do not overcook. Add cooked rice.

Creamy Carrot Soup (P)

Serves 2

10 carrots, washed and cut into 1 inch pieces

1 large sweet onion, chopped

2 cups almond milk or broth

1 tsp. fresh ginger, grated

1 clove garlic, minced

¼ cup cashews

This also makes a wonderful carrot soup without being pureed.

Add all ingredients except cashews to pot and cook on low, until carrots are tender. In increments, puree mixture in food processor or blender. Be very careful about the steam, it will blow the cover off the blender! Return to pan. Put 1 cup of pureed soup and cashews in blender, blend until nuts are creamy. Add to soup. For presentation; top soup with finely chopped cashews.

Sans Cream of Broccoli (P)

Serves 4 – 6

2 bunches broccoli, cut into florets

1 clove garlic

2 celery stalks, sliced

6 cups broth

¼ tsp. thyme

¼ tsp. bouquet garni

When ready to serve, drizzle each bowl with a bit of lemon juice if desired.

Cut broccoli into florets. Cut stems into chunks. Add all ingredients in stock pan. Bring to a boil. Lower heat to medium/low, simmer 20 – 30 minutes. Do not boil. When vegetables are tender, remove 2 cups of broccoli florets.

Add soup to blender in increments, blending until smooth. Be cautious when blending, as hot steam with blow the cover off. Return blended vegetables to pan. Add reserved broccoli florets. Serve.

If desired, garnish with sunflower or pumpkin seeds.

Butternut Squash (P)

Serves 4

1 large fresh or frozen butternut squash, peeled, cut into large chunks (about 4 cups)

5 oz. fresh spinach (1 small plastic container)

4 cups water or organic chicken broth

¼ cup almond milk

1 apple, peeled, cut

Spice/herb of choice: fennel, nutmeg, etc.

In stock pan, add squash, apple, spice of choice, and water. Cook on medium heat, covered, until squash breaks apart with fork.

Puree in blender or food processor or fork mash. Be very careful with the blender; hot steam will blow lid off. Return blended soup to pot.

Add spinach and almond milk. Turn off heat. Cover until spinach wilts.

Note: For proper food combining, substitute chicken broth for almond milk.

Green Life Minestrone Ⓟ

Serves 4 – 6

If omitting rice, reduce water to 4 ½ cups.

1 ½ cups cooked brown rice

6 cups broth, chicken or vegetable

1 cup snow peas or sugar snap peas, trimmed, cut in half

8 spears asparagus, trim ends, cut in 1-inch pieces

½ cup peas, fresh or frozen

1 clove garlic, (if permitted)

¼ – ½ tsp. spices of choice such as basil, Thai basil, sage, oregano, etc.

Add water, garlic and rice to stock pan. Bring to boil. Cover, lower heat. Simmer until rice is tender, about 35 – 45 minutes. Add vegetables and spices. Simmer approximately 5 minutes, until vegetables are al dente (cooked but crunchy).

Remember to account for any extra time the soup will sit prior to serving because vegetables will continue to cook in hot water, even with stove turned off. If vegetables are over cooked they will not stay bright green.

Note: For proper food combining use vegetable broth, not chicken broth.

Greens and Turkey Bacon (P)

Serves 4

3 strips of free range turkey bacon, chopped

32 oz. organic, low-sodium chicken broth

1 ½ Tbs. fennel seeds

1 bunch swiss chard, kale, or collard greens
or equivalent combination of greens

1 clove garlic, minced

1 bunch scallions or onions, chopped

Chop turkey bacon. Set aside. Prepare greens by tearing leaf from stem. Discard stem. Stack 4 – 6 leaves at a time, roll tightly. Starting at one end, slice into thin ribbons,. Combine all ingredients in stock pan. Cook on medium low until greens are tender, approximately 5 – 7 minutes.

Chicken Sausage Soup (P)

Serves 4

1 organic chicken sausage

32 oz. organic, low or no sodium chicken broth

1 Tbs. fennel seeds

1 – 2 bunches of swiss chard, kale, escarole, spinach, arugula (small clamshell box) or any combination

4 cloves garlic, minced

If using fresh, raw sausage, remove from casing, sauté sausage using a little broth to keep from sticking. Crumble it as it cooks. If using precooked sausage, slice lengthwise twice and chop.

For Swiss Chard and kale, remove center rib and stack leaves, roll them lengthwise and cut into thin ribbons. If using escarole or a bunch of spinach, simply chop. If using a plastic, clamshell container of arugula or spinach, either leave whole or cut smaller with a pair of scissors.

Add all ingredients to stock pot. Cook on medium heat until greens are wilted. Serve hot.

Vegetable Chicken Soup (P)

Serves 6 – 8

1 fennel bulb, trimmed, chopped (discard leafy stalks)

1 skinless, boneless chicken breast

2 cups kale, remove stems, chopped

1 medium carrot, sliced

2 cups cabbage, shredded

5 cups water or broth

10 – 12 oz. fresh or frozen green beans, cut into ½ inch pieces

2 small zucchini, chopped

2 sprigs fresh thyme

1 bay leaf

5 cups baby spinach

Topping (omit for proper food combining)

1 ½ cups fresh basil

½ cup nuts or seeds (cashews or pine nuts are creamiest)

1 tsp. olive oil

2 tsp. water

In stock pan add, chicken, fennel, kale, carrots, cabbage, water and broth. Simmer, uncovered, 30 minutes. Add green beans, squash, thyme, and bay leaf. Simmer until vegetables are tender, approximately another 10 minutes. Remove and discard thyme sprigs and bay leaf. Remove chicken, let cool. Shred by hand or chop. Return to soup. Remove soup from heat. Add spinach to hot soup. Cover pan. Allow soup to sit until spinach is wilted.

Blend all topping ingredients in blender. When serving, add a dollop of blended topping to each bowl of soup.

Meatball Vegetable Soup (P)

Serves 8

> *Hans all natural sweet basil meatballs are great. Look for low sodium meatballs.*

12 – 16 small chicken or beef meatballs, cooked

8 cups chicken, beef or vegetable broth

2 medium zucchini, cubed

3 large carrots, sliced

3 large celery stalks, sliced

1 fennel bulb, chop only the white portion

½ cup peas, fresh or frozen

2 Tbs. dried oregano

2 Tbs. dried parsley

6 – 8 cloves garlic, chopped

Add broth, carrots, fennel and celery to stock pan. Cook on medium heat until vegetables almost soft. Add meatballs, zucchini, spices, herbs and peas. Continue to cook about 10 minutes. Serve.

Top with a pesto from the Dressing, Sauces & Dips section for an added touch.

Note: Pre-made meatballs are fast and easy, or make a batch and freeze in portion sizes for a quick dinner. They can be added frozen. I like to chop the meatballs to give the appearance of more meat to those meat lovers in the family! This trick also helps to keep the weekly animal protein intake to 12 – 14 oz. per week.

Fish Chowder (P)

Recipe adapted from Amanda Harris
Serves 4

This wonderful recipe is a delicious, versatile soup. Amanda may have shared her Salmon Chowder recipe, but it easily goes far beyond! I am from New England, and clam chowder is a staple and not as tasty anywhere else. But since my awareness of clean and unclean seafood, I won't eat clams. And since I don't like salmon, I substituted with cod fish. I omitted the broccoli and added the corn, garnished with fresh parsley and it was like being in New England again eating clam chowder! For something different I use the creamed cauliflower with bacon as the base and add various fresh or frozen vegetables. I have also roasted the other half of the cauliflower and other vegetables of choice and added those in to the pureed cauliflower base. It's even fantastic with the creamed base, bacon and wilting baby spinach. This soup is always a hit.

Optional: Substitute broccoli for 1 cup of organic corn

3 cups unsweetened almond milk
½ head cauliflower, chopped
1 cup broccoli, chopped
½ cup carrots, shredded
4 slices turkey bacon, chopped
½ cup celery, chopped
3 lemon slices
2 – 3 Tbs. fresh parsley, for garnish (optional)
¼ cup onion, chopped
6 oz. salmon or clean white fish, cut in bite size chunks

In stock pan, sauté onions on medium/low heat. Use a little water to keep them from sticking. When cooked, set aside.

(Recipe continues on next page)

Combine cauliflower and almond milk in same stock pan, cook on medium until cauliflower is soft. Transfer to blender and process until smooth.

Return the blended mixture to pan. Add vegetables, fish and bacon. Cook until vegetables are tender.

Squeeze lemon slices into soup, discard rind. Add sautéed onions. Garnish with parsley. Serve.

Note: For proper food combining, substitute chicken or vegetable broth for almond milk.

Dressings, Sauces, & Dips

Dressings, Sauces, & Dips

THINK OUTSIDE THE BOTTLE! These dressings and sauces can be put on salad, chopped chicken or tuna, steamed vegetables, raw vegetables, rice or pasta. No need to fret about not having spaghetti sauce when you have these versatile sauces! Just like all recipes, think outside the box with pasta and rice. We traditionally think of putting meat or stir fry on rice, and red sauce or cream sauce on pasta, but this section offers some tasty, non-traditional toppings for rice, pasta, meats, and veggies.

A Few Tasty Tips

Many of the following recipes are based on avocado and artichokes. Avocado is ripe when the peel is darker green/black color and just gives under the pressure of your fingers. Artichoke hearts can be found jarred in water or frozen. Avoid the artichoke hearts that are marinated or in oil.

Avocado sauce is great for making chicken salad! Dip with a celery stick, cucumber or zucchini rather than crackers. If only a cracker will do then use the Brown Rice Tortilla Chips recipe in the Treats section, but remember to watch for proper food combining when dealing with gut issues.

Always keep oil to a minimum. Nuts, seeds and avocados are all fat sources. Even if they are 'good' fats, they are still fattening. If garlic is permitted, try roasted garlic as follows: peel cloves, wrap in parchment paper then foil, drizzle a bit of olive oil. Wrap tightly, bake at 375° until soft, approximately 15 – 20 minutes. Or simply put peeled cloves (whole or cut) in oven proof dish, drizzle with olive oil. Bake at 350° until soft, approximately 15 – 20 minutes. Some recipes are titled "sauce" while others are titled "dressing;" mix and match recipes for whatever you think the flavor will enhance. For example a "dressing" can be made thicker and used for a dip.

Nut Milks

If a recipe calls for almond milk or rice milk, any nut milk will be a fine substitute. If a store bought nut milk cannot be found from your permitted list, making it homemade is fast and easy. Use the Homemade Nut Milk recipe found in the Smoothies & Beverages section. Vary the amount of water according to your taste preference. The average ratio is 1 cup nuts or seeds to 2 – 3 cups water. My favorite variation is 1 cup almonds to 3 cups water with nothing else added.

Directions for Recipes

Unless otherwise specified, directions for the following recipes are as follows: simply put ingredients into a high powered blender or coffee grinder and process until smooth. Raw pine nuts, sunflower seeds, pumpkin seeds or raw macadamia nuts can be substituted for nuts listed.

Be creative! Make your own variations. For thicker consistency add nuts or avocado. Cucumber can be added for thinning because of its high water content. Just mix and match herbs with lemon or lime.

Cucumber Dressing (P)

Makes 1 cup

1 pickle-size cucumber, chopped.
or ½ English cucumber.

¼ ripe avocado, scoop out flesh

2 Tbs. fresh lemon juice

1 Tbs. fresh dill, chopped

1 Tbs. fresh cilantro, chopped

1 clove garlic, minced

Creamy Herb Dressing (P)

Makes 1 cup

4 – 8 cloves garlic, roasted
(see directions at beginning of section)
or 2 – 3 fresh cloves garlic, minced

1 cup unsweetened almond or rice milk

½ cup sunflower butter,
or make other nut butter from raw nuts or seeds in blender

2 Tbs. fresh lemon juice or juice of 2 limes

Spices/herbs of choice such as rosemary, basil,
tarragon, parsley, cilantro, oregano, etc.

Garlicky Lemon Dressing (P)

Makes ½ cup

2 cloves garlic, minced

5 tablespoons pine nuts or cashews

3 teaspoons fresh lemon juice

1 teaspoon olive oil

½ teaspoon lemon zest

Add water while blending to reach desired consistency.

Kob Farms House Dressing (M)

Recipe by Kelly Marra, RawLifeCoaching.com

Makes 3 ½ cups

This dressing is amazing! In my house, we use it on everything, from salads to a dip for veggie sticks and even as a replacement for any creamy dairy sauce.

¾ cup Thai coconut water

2 cloves garlic, peeled

½ cup lemon juice

1 ½ tsp. salt

1 ¼ cup raw cashews

¼ cup stone-ground mustard

2 Tbs. herbs such as parsley, basil, dill or a combination

Creamy Avocado and Herb Dressing (P)

Makes 1 ½ cups

4 – 8 cloves garlic, roasted
(see directions at beginning of section)

1 cup unsweetened almond or rice milk

1 avocado

2 Tbs. fresh lemon juice or juice of 2 limes

Spices/herbs of choice such as rosemary, basil, tarragon, parsley, cilantro, oregano

Creamy Lemony Dressing (P)

Makes ½ cup

2 cloves garlic, minced

5 Tbs. raw pine nuts or raw macadamia nuts

3 tsp. fresh lemon juice

1 tsp. olive oil

½ tsp. lemon zest

Add water while blending to reach desired consistency.

Tangy Cashew Dressing (P)

Makes ½ cup

1 cup raw cashews

1 small clove garlic

zest of one lemon

4 – 5 Tbs. fresh lemon juice

¼ cup filtered water
or substitute an equal amount of cucumber
(peeled or un-peeled) that has been blended into a liquid

Variations
- *1 cup almond milk*
- *1 cup raw cashews*
- *½ cup Riesling Raisin Vinegar*

Sunshine Dressing (M)

Makes 1 ½ cups

2 oranges, peeled and seeded

⅓ cup raw cashews

2 – 3 Tbs. of Blood Orange vinegar

Berrylicious Dressing (P)

Makes ½ cup

1 cup berries

¼ cup water

¼ cup raw cashews

1 ½ Tbs. fruit infused vinegar

Light Raisin Dressing (M)

Makes 1 cup

1 small English cucumber or medium regular cucumber, seeded

½ cup raisins or currants

¼ cup raw almond butter or raw cashew butter

2 tsp. Riesling Raisin vinegar

Variations

- *1 cup almond milk*
- *1 cup raw cashews*
- *½ cup Riesling Raisin Vinegar*

Apple Nut Butter Dressing (P)

Makes 1 cup

2 Tbs. almond butter

⅓ cup almond or rice milk

1 apple, cored, chopped

¼ tsp. vanilla (optional)

Apple Tahini Dressing (P)

Makes 3 cups

2 cups almond or rice milk

1 cup fresh apple, seeded, cubed

⅓ cup raw tahini (pureed sesame seeds)

2 Tbs. unhulled sesame seeds

¼ cup water

Green Velvet Dressing/Dip (P)

Makes 1 cup

¾ cup water

½ cup fresh lemon juice

½ cup raw tahini

¼ cup fresh parsley, chopped

¼ cup fresh dill, chopped

4 Tbs. raw cashews, macadamia nuts or pine nuts

½ Tbs. fresh tarragon, chopped (optional)

2 cloves garlic, minced

Fresh Cucumber Dip (M)

Recipe by Kelly Marra, RawLifeCoaching.com

Makes 1 ½ Cups

This dip is perfect for summer. Cucumbers can really cool you off!

½ cup raw cashews,
soaked in water for 20 minutes

1 cucumber, peeled

½ avocado

1 tsp. olive oil

2 Tbs. dried dill

Drain and rinse cashew with fresh water. Put all ingredients in a blender and blend well. Taste and adjust seasonings to personal preference. Enjoy on sandwiches, crackers, wraps, and with veggie sticks.

Artichoke Sauce/Dip (P)

Makes 3 – 4

This recipe will make enough sauce for approximately 4 servings of pasta, rice or vegetables. Reduce ingredients for smaller batches. If a thinner sauce is desired, add peeled cucumber due to its high water content or just omit avocado, which makes the sauce thick and creamy.

4 jars artichoke hearts, jarred in water or frozen, defrosted

4 – 6 cloves garlic, roasted until soft

8 Tbs. fresh basil, chopped fine

4 Tbs. fresh parsley, chopped fine

juice 1 fresh lemon, add in increments and taste

1 avocado

Mix artichoke hearts, garlic and avocado in blender. Process until smooth or left slightly chunky. Mix in herbs and lemon juice by hand. Toss into hot pasta or rice, mix with cooked vegetables or use for dip with raw vegetables. Best if all ingredients are at room temperature; the heat of the food will slightly the heat the sauce. If a hotter sauce if preferred, blend artichokes and garlic only. Heat on stove top. Mash avocado by hand, add herbs then mix avocado mixture by hand into heated sauce. Only use avocado if serving immediately as it will oxidize and does not reheat well.

Note: To roast such a small portion of garlic, peel cloves, put a few drops of olive oil, wrap in foil and roast at 400° for 10 – 15 minutes until soft.

Optional:
Steam or roast ½ head of cauliflower, mix in blender until smooth then follow the directions above for blending artichokes, etc. If using the cauliflower, omit avocado.

Artichoke Sunflower Spread Ⓟ

Makes about 1 – 1½ cups

½ cup raw, hulled sunflower seeds

1 package frozen artichoke hearts (9 oz.), defrosted
or 1 jar drained (jarred in water)

2 cloves garlic, peeled

1 Tbs. olive oil

1 tsp. fresh oregano
or ¼ tsp. dried oregano

Raw pumpkin seeds may be substituted for sunflower seeds. Soak seeds in warm, filtered water several hours. Drain.

Process in blender or food processor until smooth. Add artichoke hearts and garlic, continue blending until smooth. Finally, add olive oil, and oregano. Blend until smooth.

Super Healthy Guacamole Dip Ⓟ

Recipe by Kelly Marra, RawLifeCoaching.com

Serves 4

2 avocados

6 cups spinach, packed

1 Tbs. lime juice

¼ cup cilantro (optional)

1 ½ tsp salt

Peel and pit the avocados. Put avocado, spinach, lime juice, cilantro and salt in a food processor, process until very smooth. Stop to scrape down the sides of the food processor if necessary and process again. Enjoy on crackers, chips, sandwiches or on veggie sticks.

Avocado Sauce/Dip (P)

Serves 4

2 ripe avocados

¼ cup unsweetened almond milk

½ cup fresh basil, chopped

juice ½ fresh lemon

Spice or herb of choice such as
rosemary, oregano, cilantro

For dip, omit almond milk. Experiment with different spices/herbs. Try adding chopped olives.

Heat the rice milk in a small saucepan. Put remaining ingredients in blender. Add warm rice milk, in small increments, blending until desired consistency. For a chunky consistency, use a potato masher instead of the blender.

Avo-Choke Sauce/Dip (P)

Makes 1 ½ cups

1 jar artichoke hearts, drained
(packed in water not oil)

1 ripe avocado

1 Tbs. lemon juice, add in increments and taste

Spice or herb of choice such as
basil, parsley, rosemary, oregano, cilantro

Adjust the thickness of the sauce by adjusting the quantity of avocado. For example, if a thinner sauce is desired, omit some avocado. If a thicker sauce is desired, add more avocado.

Pasta Sauce (P)

Serves 2 – 3

1 zucchini squash

1 yellow squash

2 carrots

½ head cauliflower

8 cloves garlic

¼ cup fresh basil, chopped

1 Tbs. fresh parsley, chopped

1 - 2 cups water or broth, if needed for thinner sauce

Preheat oven to 450°. Roast vegetables according to directions for Roasted Vegetables in Vegetables section. Unpeeled garlic cloves can be added to cookie sheet and cooked until soft. Add roasted vegetables to blender in increments. Blend until smooth, adding fresh parsley. Add mixture to sauce pan. Simmer until heated. Serve over pasta, rice or cooked vegetables.

For faster sauce, sauté or steam all vegetables. Mince raw garlic. Blend vegetables with minced garlic. Add to sauce pan with chopped herbs. Simmer until garlic is cooked.

Natural sugars are brought out in roasted vegetables so the flavor will be different from steamed or sautéed vegetables.

If sauce is too thick, thin out by adding water or broth.

White Sauce (P)

Makes 1 ½ cups

1 Tbs. olive oil

3 Tbs. brown rice flour
(make fresh by grinding brown rice in coffee grinder)

1 ½ cups rice milk

spice/herb of choice

In pot, add rice milk and spices/herbs. Simmer on low. Add flour and 1 cup of warm milk to tightly covered jar. Shake vigorously to blend without lumps or put in blender.

Add oil to warmed sauce prior to serving. Serve over cooked vegetables such as asparagus or cooked brown rice pasta.

Basil Pesto (P)

Makes about 1 ½ cups

2 cloves garlic, peeled

⅓ cup pine nuts (may substitute other nuts or seeds)

2 cups fresh basil, lightly packed

¼ cup olive oil

1 ½ – 3 tsp. fresh squeezed lemon juice (optional)

1 artichoke heart, frozen and defrosted
or jarred in water (optional)

In blender or food processor, combine garlic and nuts. Blend. Add basil and olive oil, blending until basil is finely chopped.

Cilantro Pesto (P)

Makes about 1 cup

3 cups fresh cilantro, tightly packed

¼ cup raw cashew, macadamia or pine nuts

2 cloves garlic

¼ cup olive oil

1 Tbs. fresh lemon juice

In food processor or blender, combine cilantro, nuts, juice and garlic. Process until smooth. With machine running, add olive oil. Process into a smooth paste.

Mint Pesto (P)

Makes about 1 ½ cups

⅓ cup almonds
(may substitute other permitted nuts or seeds)

2 cups fresh mint, tightly packed

¼ cup olive oil

½ – 1 Tbs. fresh squeezed lemon juice
(optional)

In blender or food processor, blend nuts. Add mint, lemon juice and olive oil. Blend until mint is finely chopped. Start with adding only ½ tablespoon lemon juice, adjusting to taste as needed.

Olive Pate ⓟ

Makes 2 cups

1 cup Kalamata olives, pitted

1 cup canned black olives

1 clove garlic, minced

2 Tbs. raw pine nuts

1 Tbs. fresh parsley, chopped

1 Tbs. extra-virgin olive oil

Put all ingredients in a food processor or blender on low. Blend until ingredients are chopped finely but still have visible pieces.

Smoothies & Beverages

Smoothies & Beverages

These smoothie creations are limited only by your imagination! While on the program, you are limited to peaches, pears, plums and apples; however, there are still a great variety of choices. Technically, mixing fruit and greens is not a proper food combination. However, most people are able to enjoy smoothies. Smoothies are great for breakfast or a pre-breakfast drink. As a pre-breakfast drink, wait a ½ hour before eating breakfast. Smoothies are also perfect for a fast snack or pick me up before reaching for a cookie or coffee. Smoothies make it easy to get greens into kids, even big kids! Don't be intimidated by adding greens; baby lettuce leaves and spinach are virtually tasteless when added to a smoothie. Experiment with ingredients. If you find a smoothies too thick, add more liquid or ice to thin it out and save some for a snack later in the day. Smoothies will freeze well, so you can make them in batches and freeze in individual "to go" containers so you can grab one as you're running out the door.

Beverages on the program do not include the Standard American Diet choices of coffee, tea, soda, juice or alcohol. The programs' primary beverages are water and caffeine-free tea. So for those folks who don't enjoy water, I have included some recipes that I created out of my imagination and others I have experienced elsewhere. The average water consumption rule is half your body weight in ounces. While hard-core believers in the "rule" will disagree with me, I believe that freshly flavored water and nut milks count toward your total water intake. Water is the most healthy beverage of choice, but adding some zip is fun and tasty.

Notes on Smoothies & Beverages

Smoothies

Directions for these smoothies are all the same: put all ingredients in a high powered blender, process on high until smooth. Ice or frozen fruit can be added for a thick icy smoothie. Frozen fruit will substitute nicely for fresh fruit. Saluté!

Beverages

As mentioned at the beginning of this section, water is the beverage of choice. Tea is permitted but it must be caffeine free, not decaffeinated. Decaffeinated tea and coffee still contain caffeine. The recipes included here are for flavored water for folks who get tired of drinking "plain ole" water. Even though citrus is added in the waters, it is still not permitted for eating.

Nut milks are great for straight up drinking, baking, smoothies and dressings. A word of caution on the nuts, they are high in fat, so moderation is key while on the weight loss program. Nut milks can also be warmed slightly. Since they are made with raw nuts, do not over heat them or the enzymes will be destroyed. Nut milks can be strained with a good old flour sifter or through cheese cloth for a finer liquid. Just place the sifter over a large mouth jar or large glass measuring cup, or secure the cheese cloth with a rubber band around the mouth of the jar or container, and pour slowly. I use the sifter method and make fresh nut milk in 5 minutes. Store nut milks in a sealed container or jar in fridge for up to 4 days. Nut pulp will settle to the bottom of the container, so pouring slowly will keep out even more pulp.

Apple Pie (P)

Serves 1

1 large apple, quartered

¼ cup walnuts

5 oz. baby spinach or baby greens

1 tsp. cinnamon

¼ tsp. vanilla

1 ½ cups unsweetened almond or rice milk

Apple-Cado (P)

Serves 1

1 apple, quartered

½ avocado, peeled and pitted

5 – 8 oz. organic baby spinach

½ cup liquid

Ap-a-cado (with Dates) (M)

Serves 1

1 apple

½ avocado, peeled and pitted

1 – 2 pitted dates

5 oz. organic baby spinach

½ cup liquid

Creamy Peach (P)

Serves 1

2 fresh peaches, pitted

½ cup liquid

2 ice cubes

1 tsp. almond butter

Substitute fresh peaches with 1 ½ – 2 cups frozen peaches, omit ice and add ½ cup water.

Fruit & Nutty (P)

Serves 1

1 cup liquid

1 apple, cored and cut

5 – 6 oz. greens, baby spinach, baby romaine or mixed greens

1 heaping Tbs. raw almond butter

Bob's Very Berry Beet Smoothie (M)

Recipe by Bob Willix

Serves 1

½ cup blueberries

1 organic carrot

1 organic apple

1 raw beet, peeled and cut into chunks

3 kale leaves

1 cup ice

A Vitamix blender is recommended for this recipe.

Note: For proper food combining, substitute apple instead of blueberries.

Vegetable Smoothie Ⓟ

Serves 1

3 – 5 oz. greens

1 celery stalk

½ cucumber, cut in large chunks

1 apple, quartered

1 cup liquid

Green Power Ⓟ

Serves 1

6 – 8 oz. organic spinach

1 cup liquid

1 avocado

1 Tbs. raw tahini

1 Tbs. lemon juice

Zippy Smoothie I Ⓟ

Serves 1

1 apple or pear

6 – 8 leaves romaine lettuce

⅓ cup fresh, flat parsley

½ avocado

juice ½ lemon

1 cup water

Zippy Smoothie II (P)

Serves 1

1 apple or pear

6 – 8 leaves romaine lettuce or 2 handfuls baby spinach

⅓ cup fresh, flat parsley

¼ cup fresh mint

½ avocado

⅔ English cucumber

⅓ cup fresh aloe vera leaf, peeled

juice of ½ lemon

1 cup water

Super Smoothie (M)

Serves 2

¼ cup raw pepitas (pumpkin seeds),
pine nuts, almonds, walnuts or nut/seed of choice

1 Tbs. chia seed

¼ cup cooked, cold oats, quinoa, millet,
brown rice or buckwheat

4- 6 ounces leafy greens

1 avocado

2 cups any combination apples, pears and/or peaches

1 cup liquid

Drink immediately as chia seeds will turn gelatinous.

'Hot' Oatmeal Smoothie (M)

Serves 1

1 cup liquid

3 Tbs. cooked hot steel cut oats, old-fashioned oatmeal, or short-grain brown rice

1 apple, peach or pear, chopped (not peeled)

1 ounce raw nuts

¼ teaspoon cinnamon

Homemade Nut Milk (P)

Serves 1

1 cup raw nuts

3 cups filtered water

1 ½ teaspoons vanilla or one vanilla bean (optional)

1– 2 Tbs. approved sweetener (optional)

If you have a dehydrator, the leftover almond pulp can be dehydrated then ground into almond flour.

To spice it up, add ½ tsp. pumpkin spice, nutmeg, or cardamom. Blend all ingredients and strain through a fine sieve such as a flour sifter, cheese cloth, or panty hose.

Apple Nut Milk (P)

Serves 1

⅓ cup raw nuts

⅔ cup apple, cut

3 cups filtered water

Peach Nut Milk (P)

Serves 1

⅓ cup raw nuts

2 fresh peaches, cut

3 cups filtered water

Nutnog/Seednog (P)

Serves 1

1 cup raw nuts or seeds

2 cups water

½ tsp. nutmeg

1 – 2 Tbs. acceptable sweetener

1 ½ tsp. vanilla extract
or one pliable vanilla bean with center scraped out

dash of cinnamon

Soak nuts a few hours or over night. Put ingredients in high powered blender, process until nuts are thoroughly ground. Add water until you reach desired consistency. Depending on desired smoothness, milk can be enjoyed with pulp or strained through a fine mesh sieve. Discard strained pulp.

Orange Creamsicle (P)

Makes 1 gallon

1 gallon filtered water

1 navel orange, washed well, sliced into thin rings

1 pliable, vanilla bean, cut lengthwise into 2 pieces

Fill gallon jug with filtered water, but not to capacity. Leave room for water to rise when adding remaining ingredients. Add remaining ingredients. Refrigerate 24 hours before serving.

Fruity Iced Tea Cooler (P)

Serves 1

1 cup caffeine free tea

½ - ¾ cups frozen peaches

Alternate recipe

1 cup caffeine free tea

1 apple, pear or peach, cut

5-6 ice cubes, or cubes of frozen tea

Put all ingredients in high powered blender, blending until smooth. With some blenders, additional liquid may be needed.

Ruby Red Cucumber (P)

Makes 1 gallon

1 gallon filtered water

1 ruby red grapefruit, washed well, sliced into thin rings

1 cucumber, peeled and thinly sliced

Fill gallon jug with filtered water, but not to capacity; leave room for water to rise when adding remaining ingredients. Add remaining ingredients. Refrigerate 24 hours before serving.

Treats... Oh, Yes!

Treats... Oh, Yes!

Deprivation is never pleasant, especially when it comes to our goodies. Moderation, of course, is still key when indulging in items from this section. These treats can be enjoyed as a snack or breakfast. Technically, some do not follow proper food combining guidelines. But depending on the state of your personal digestive health, these infractions should be okay. Another word of caution; fruit becomes acidic when cooked. Since healing the gut is so important to the success of this program there are a few things here that will hinder that process, so be very careful with these indulgences. Muffins are a standard for the Standard American Diet but their listing here does not make them a standard on this plan; it merely makes it an option for an occasional treat. Balance is the rule here.

If you have a high powered blender it is possible to make your own nut flours and rice flours. A coffee grinder actually does a fine job as well. Just add the dry, whole grains or nuts and blend until a flour consistency. Don't get hooked on nut butters, especially while on the weight loss program. Nut butters are high in fat, which of course brings them into the delicious but dangerous zone. Here's to feeling decadent!

Agar Agar vs. Gelatin

Agar Agar is not your grandmother's Jello! Agar agar is thought of as the "vegetarian gelatin." It is derived from South East Asian seaweed and means 'jelly.'

Agar Agar can be found in flakes, whole strands or powder. If using the whole strands, place in coffee grinder to reduce to flakes. If you don't have a food processor or Vitamix then purchase the flakes or powder. One teaspoon of Agar Agar powder is equivalent to one tablespoon of flakes. It is important to add ingredients (such as fruits) into the pan of dissolved Agar and cook it gently. This step is important for two reasons; some fruits have enzymes that inhibit the Agar from firming up and when cold ingredients are added it will firm up faster. So, don't add cold items until you are ready for it to set.

When creating your own recipes if it is too thick or too thin, put it back into a pan and add more liquid or more Agar Agar. Amazingly, it melts back down when heated so errors can be corrected. However, if adding more Agar is necessary, I suggest mixing it with a little water, heating until completely dissolved then adding in the mixture to melt down. This insures the Agar is completely dissolved. If converting a recipe that calls for gelatin, the same amount of powdered Agar Agar can be substituted for powdered gelatin.

So why would you want to substitute Agar for gelatin? Gelatin comes from animals; so vegans and vegetarians would not likely consume gelatin products. But even some carnivores find the source less than appealing. Gelatin is made by boiling bones, hooves, skin and tendons of various animals, basically the discard of the meat industry.

A Note About Sweeteners

Follow the guide below when replacing dry sweeteners with liquid sweeteners and vise versa.

- 1 cup dry with 1 cup liquid: reduce any liquid by ⅓ cup or add 4 – 5 Tbs. flour to dry ingredients
- 1 cup dry with ¾ cups honey: reduce any liquid by ¼ cup or add ⅓ cup flour to dry ingredients
- 1 cup liquid with 1 cup dry: add ⅓ cup water or nut milk
- 1 cup liquid with ¾ cups honey: add ¼ cup water or nut milk

Almond Flour Muffins Ⓜ

Makes 12 muffins

2 cups almond flour (almond meal)

2 Tbs. aluminum-free baking powder

¼ tsp. salt

½ cup raw apple, peeled, grated and packed (Golden delicious, preferred)

4 eggs (may substitute 8 yolks or 8 whites)

⅓ cup filtered water

⅓ cup allowed natural sweetener

Preheat oven to 350°. Oil a 12-cup muffin tin. Mix all ingredients together. If batter bubbles, stir down before filling muffin tins. Ignore the usual directions for mixing muffins (to fold liquid and dry ingredients together until just moistened). Beat well (no "tunnels" form when using almond meal). Transfer batter to muffin tins filling ¾ to ⅞ full. Bake for approximately 18 – 20 minutes. For miniature muffins, bake 15 minutes. Muffins are done when a toothpick inserted comes out clean.

Quinoa Flour Muffins (M)

Makes 12 muffins

1½ cups quinoa flour

½ cup tapioca flour

1 tsp. aluminum-free baking powder

½ tsp. sea salt

1 egg (may substitute with 2 whites or 2 yolks)

⅓ cup coconut oil

1 cup rice milk

Preheat over to 400°. Mix dry and wet ingredients separately. Fold together quickly, but gently, until just blended. Do not over mix. Fill oiled muffin cups ½ full. Bake 12 – 15 minutes or until nicely browned. For mini muffins bake at 375° for 20 minutes.

Variations

- *Almond meal or other nut meal may be substituted for quinoa flour.*
- *Use unsweetened almond milk in place of rice milk.*

Rice Flour Muffins (M)

Makes 12 muffins

2 cups brown rice flour

2 tsp. aluminum-free baking powder

1 egg, beaten

4 Tbs., liquid natural sweetener

1 Tbs. olive oil

1 tsp. vanilla extract

1 cup rice milk

Preheat oven to 350°. Lightly oil a dozen 2 ½ inch muffin tins. Mix dry and liquid ingredients separately. Add dry ingredients to liquids, gently whisk together until just mixed. Divide batter equally between all 12 muffin tins (filling approximately ¾ full). Batter will be runny. Bake 28 minutes, until lightly browned. Remove from pan onto rack to cool.

Homemade Granola (P)

Makes 3 cups

3 cups old fashioned oats

1 ½ cups various permitted nuts and/or seeds

¼ cup permitted sweetener

¼ cup coconut oil

1 tsp. vanilla

Note: For proper food combining, omit nuts/seeds.

Preheat oven to 350°. Combine oats with nuts/seeds in bowl. In separate bowl, combine remaining ingredients. Mix. Combine both mixtures together. Spread mixture in thin layer on large baking sheet. Bake approximately 45 minutes. Stir granola every 10 minutes to insure even browning. Cool. Store in airtight container.

Cashew Cream (P)

Makes ½ – ¾ cups

½ cup raw cashews
(always use raw nuts)

3 Tbs. filtered water

1 pitted date (optional for sweetness)

nutmeg, cinnamon, pumpkin spice or vanilla
(optional, add a tiny bit at a time and taste)

I don't usually add anything but the nuts and water. Nut creams can be made with almost any nut. The creamiest will be cashews, pine nuts and macadamia nuts because of the fat content. Always use raw nuts.

The trick is to start with the least amount of water and work up for the consistency of a firm cream, not runny. I find the Bullet or coffee grinder works best. The only blender I know that can do a good job is the Vitamix, but it's hard to make only a little bit and then try to get it out of the blender.

Add all the ingredients at the same time and blend, adding water as it processes, until desired consistency. Don't make the mistake of adding water to fast, the Bullet and grinder will sound like they don't have enough liquid and are struggling, give it time.

Note: To make this recipe program compliant, omit dates.

This makes a great topping for muffins. No need to use fancy baking tools – just put the cream in a plastic bag, pressing it all to one corner. Snip the corner and squeeze out the cream. A little dollop is a beautiful presentation on the mini muffins. For regular sized muffins, cut out a small cone-shaped piece from the center of the muffin and fill the hole with cream. Replace the muffin piece on top.

Nutty Dippin' Ⓟ

Use any raw nut or seed butter:

Stuff celery stalks or dip celery into nut butter

Cut apples or pears into wedges and dip

Slice cucumbers or zucchini into spears and dip

Nut Butter Wraps Ⓟ

Makes 4 – 6

1 full head romaine lettuce, not romaine hearts

raw nut butter

carrot, shredded

apple, shredded

cinnamon, sprinkled

Remove hard end of lettuce, layer 2 lettuce leaves together, placing end to end with ends at opposite sides. For smaller inside leaves, use 3 leaves. Spread nut butter down center of leaf. Top with remaining ingredients. Roll lengthwise. Eat like burrito. Or, if rolling from top to bottom, press stem with thumbs to break it a bit, roll, starting at stem end of outside leaf.

Caramelized Brown Rice Pudding (M)

Serves 4

4 cups (1 quart) rice milk, unsweetened
2 cups brown rice, cooked
¼ cup raisins (optional)
1 tsp. each cinnamon, nutmeg, and vanilla
1 cups rice milk, unsweetened
2 eggs, beaten

I prefer currants over raisin because they are smaller and not so over-powering. Another favorite option is using chopped fresh peaches.

Caramelize 4 cups rice milk by heating over low heat to reduce to around 1 cup in volume over very low heat. This may take several hours. Rice milk will turn color (light caramel color) and just start to thicken.

Remove from heat. Add rest of ingredients except eggs and vanilla, stirring well. By adding eggs and vanilla last, mixture will then be cool enough that the eggs will not curdle.

Return to very low heat setting for 30 minutes. Set timer and stir once or twice to make sure mixture is not sticking. Transfer pudding to a quart-size casserole and bake at 350° for approximately 40 minutes, or until set. Serve warm or cold.

Note: If you are unable to have eggs, no worries. I have made this recipe successfully without eggs.

Baked Brown Rice Pudding (M)

Serves 6

1 ½ cups organic brown rice

3 cups filtered water

¼ tsp. sea salt

2 Tbs. arrowroot powder

1 Tbs. ground cinnamon

1 ½ cups coconut milk

¼ cup maple syrup

¼ cup raisins

vanilla extract to taste (optional)

Preheat the oven to 350°. Bring the brown rice and 3 cups of filtered water to a boil in a medium saucepan. Once it is boiling, reduce heat to low. Cover and simmer for 40 – 50 minutes, or until the rice is very soft. In a large bowl, dissolve the arrowroot powder in 1 cup of the coconut milk. Then add the rice, raisins, maple syrup, cinnamon, and salt. Mix well. Pour the mixture into a large greased baking dish. Cover and bake for 1 hour, or until lightly brown and bubbly.

Remove from the oven and stir in the remaining ½ cup of coconut milk. Leave the pudding to cool for about 1 hour before serving.

Note: To make this recipe program compliant, omit the raisins and substitute rice milk for coconut milk.

Baked Peaches with Nut Cream (M)

Serves 6

Baked Peaches

6 medium peaches, peeled, sliced

1 ½ – 2 cups granola mix,
get the lowest sugar content
or make your own

½ – 1 cup permitted nuts, chopped

Peaches may be substituted with pears or apples.

Preheat oven to 350°. Layer sliced peaches in baking dish, top with granola and nuts. Bake approximately 10 minutes, just until fruit is soft.

Nut Cream

½ – 1 cup unsweetened almond milk

1 cup permitted nuts
or ½ cup raw nut butter

¼ teaspoon vanilla

If concerned with weight gain, omit nut cream due to its high fat content.

In coffee grinder or high powered blender, combine almond milk and nuts in increments of ¼ cup almond milk add ¼ cup of nuts or 2 tablespoons of nut butter, blending each time. Increase the amount of almond milk slowly, up to 1 cup total, to reach desired consistency. Top peaches with a dollop of nut cream. Cream will keep refrigerated for several days.

Baked Fruit Bowl (M)

Serves 4

2 apples, peaches or pears, cut in half

½ cup nuts, chopped

dash cinnamon, nutmeg or cardamom, to taste

Can be topped with a nut cream from Dressings section.

Preheat oven to 350°. Use all the same fruit or any combination. Cut fruit in half, remove seeds and discard. Hollow out fruit, leaving about ¼ inch on sides and bottom. Chop scooped out fruit, mix with chopped nuts. Fill cavity of each fruit with mixture. Put in baking dish. Cover. Bake approximately 10 – 15 minutes, until fruit is tender.

Fruit Kabobs (P)

Serves 3

1 fresh peach

1 fresh apple

1 fresh pear

½ tsp. coconut oil

1 tsp. liquid sweetener

cinnamon, nutmeg or cardamom, to taste

Preheat grill to medium-high. Cut fresh peaches, apples or pears into quarters. Use all one fruit or any combination. Mix coconut oil with sweetener. Baste skewered fruit. Sprinkle with cinnamon, nutmeg or cardamom.

Grill until just tender. Serve topped with nut cream from Dressings section. Fruit can also be sliced in half, cored, dressed and grilled, cut side down.

Fruit & Oat Cobbler Ⓜ

Serves 4 – 6

4 apples, peaches, pears, chopped

2 cups granola,
use lowest in sugar or homemade

½ cup walnuts, chopped

1 teaspoon cinnamon (optional)

½ teaspoon nutmeg (optional)

Preheat oven to 350°. Combine all ingredients except fruit. Mix well. Stir in fruit. You can use all of one fruit or any combination of the three. Bake approximately 20 minutes, or until reaching desired tenderness of fruit.

Pear Crisp (P)

Serves 6 – 8

Filling

½ cup apple juice

1 Tbs. lemon juice, freshly squeezed

1 Tbs. arrowroot powder

1 tsp. ground nutmeg

5 medium pears, peeled, cored, and sliced ¼ inch thick

Use soft, fully ripened pears—Anjou, Bartlett, or Bosc work very well.

Topping

2 cups almond flour

½ tsp. sea salt

1 tsp. ground cinnamon

½ tsp. ground nutmeg

¼ cup oil

¼ cup maple syrup

1 Tbs. vanilla extract

Preheat the oven to 350°. Set aside an 8-inch square baking dish. Whisk together the apple juice, lemon juice, arrowroot powder, and nutmeg in a small bowl. Place the pears in a bowl, toss with the apple juice mixture, then transfer to the baking dish.

Combine all topping ingredients. Spread over pears. Bake uncovered about 30 minutes or until pears are soft when pierced with a fork.

Poached Pears Ⓜ

Serves 4

> *For a special touch, top with a nut cream from the Baked Peaches with the Cashew Cream recipe.*

4 pears, peeled, cored and quartered

2 cups unsweetened cranberry juice

2 cinnamon sticks

3 whole cloves

zest of ½ organic orange

walnuts, pecans, almond or nut of choice, chopped

Put all ingredients into a large saucepan. Be sure the pan is not too large, so the juice completely covers the pears. Bring to a simmer over medium heat and cook for 7 – 10 minutes. Pears should pierce easily with a fork.

To make syrup, transfer pears to a bowl. Simmer the poaching liquid until it is reduced by one third and thickened to desired consistency, 30 – 40 minutes. Pears can be stored in poaching liquid in a covered container in the refrigerator for up to 3 days. Top with chopped nuts or nut cream before serving. Can be reheated or eaten cold.

Pear-Apple Sauce Ⓟ

Serves 4 – 6

4 cups apple, chopped

1 ½ cups pear, chopped

¼ cup filtered water

½ cup nuts, chopped (optional)

Place all ingredients in saucepan. Cook covered on low until bubbling. Turn heat to low, keep covered. Cook approximately 30 – 45 minutes, depending on ripeness of fruit. Stir occasionally. Fruit is cooked when it breaks apart easily. For thinner sauce, put in blender until smooth. For chunky sauce, leave as is or fork mash to desired consistency. Top with chopped nuts. Serve warm or cold.

Stuffed Apple Ⓜ

Serves 6

> *Experiment with different varieties and sizes of apples.*

6 small apples of choice

2 cups old-fashioned oats

¼ cup liquid
(unsweetened almond milk, rice milk or water)

dash cinnamon and/or nutmeg

2 – 3 cups raw almond butter

½ cup nuts, chopped

Cut top off apples, hollow out center of apple, leaving about ¼ inch of apple to avoid puncturing through apple skin. Discard stem and seeds but save and chop scooped apple.

Place chopped apple in bowl. Add remaining ingredients. Mix well. Alter amounts of ingredients according to taste preferences. Consistency of mixture should be moist but firmly sticky and easily held together in a ball. Stuff each apple shell, wrap tightly with plastic wrap. Refrigerate.

Can be made ahead and stored in the refrigerator for 3 – 4 days.

Apple Bread(less) Pudding Ⓜ

Serves 9 – 12

> *Place oats in Vitamix, high powered blender or coffee grinder to make oat flour.*

¼ cup egg whites

¼ cup maple syrup or honey

½ lemon, peeled and seeded

4 apples, quartered

½ cup dates

¼ tsp. nutmeg

1 tsp. ground cinnamon

½ tsp. sea salt

½ tsp. aluminum free baking powder

1 cup oat flour

2 cups rolled oats

½ cup walnuts, chopped

2 Tbs. maple syrup

Preheat oven to 350°. In order listed, place egg whites, maple syrup or honey, lemon, apples, dates, nutmeg and cinnamon into Vitamix or very high powered blender. Blend on high for 1 – 2 minutes. Stop and push ingredients down if necessary or use tamper for Vitamix.

Place flour, oats, salt and baking powder in large mixing bowl, combine. Pour liquid mixture into bowl, mix. Pour into 9" x 9" baking dish. Mix walnuts with maple syrup. Pour over mixture. Bake 45 minutes. Top with vanilla cashew cream when serving.

20 Minute Fruit Pie (M)

Recipe by Kelly Marra, RawLifeCoaching.com
Makes 1 large pie

Traditional pies take forever to make, with the crust having to pre-bake and then cool off before you can add a delicious filling. This one is easy, quick and healthy!

Crust:
3 cups almonds
1 ½ cups dates, pitted and soaked in water for 20 minutes

Filling:
2 – 3 quarts fresh, ripe fruit
½ cup amber agave nectar
A squirt of fresh lemon or lime juice (optional)

Place almonds in a food processor and blend until the almonds resemble a fine powder. Drain the dates, and add them to the food processor. Process again until the dates are well incorporated. Press the mixture evenly into a pie pan.

Wash and dry the ripe fruit of your choice. Amazing fillings include: strawberries, peaches, nectarines, pineapple, mango, apples, blueberries, raspberries or blackberries. Be creative, use one fruit or a combination of fruit. Slice fruit very thin or use a fork or spoon to mash berries. Place fruit in a bowl and mix gently with agave nectar, add the optional lemon or lime juice. (If using apples, definitely add lemon or lime juice to prevent the apples from browning). Spoon fruit into the prepared pie crust, packing the fruit down with the back of the spoon. Keep adding fruit until the pie is filled to the top of the crust. Enjoy right away or chill in refrigerator.

Tropical Panna Cotta Pie (M)

Makes 8

Crust

½ cup raw walnuts

½ cup raw almonds

11 Medjool dates

or about 20 smaller dates

Experiment with nuts of choice, but always use raw nuts.

Filling

2 cups coconut milk

1 cup filtered water

1 cup fresh mango, chopped

1 cup fresh pineapple, chopped

2 Tbs. Agar Agar flakes

¼ cup amber agave nectar (optional)

fresh strawberries or bananas for garnish (optional)

For Crust: Mix all ingredients in food processor until finely minced. It should stick together easily. Put into pie plate and press into place. Set aside in refrigerator.

For Filling: Place water and flakes in saucepan. Heat on medium high, stirring frequently, it is critical to dissolve the agar completely. Add coconut milk, fruit and agave, heat. Agave is optional depending on the sweetness of the fruit. Depending on personal preference, fruit can be placed in blender until a 'crushed' consistency. Let cool. If it starts to set on the top before it has cooled, stir mixture. When cool, pour into pie plate. Return to refrigerator until completely set, about 30 – 45 minutes. Garnish with optional fruit before serving.

(Recipe continues on next page.)

Try different fruits and also try pureeing the fruits. I have noticed that by the second and third day the filling seems to develop a mild 'grainy' texture.

To make a more traditional Panna Cotta, fill ramekins with the filling and top with a berry coulis or fresh chopped fruit.

Pineapple Coconut Not-Jello (M)

Serves 4 – 6

Pick pineapples labeled "Gold" since they are the sweetest.

- 2 cups pineapple juice (see directions below)
- 5 tsp. Agar Agar flakes (found in health food stores or Asian markets)
- 1 cup fresh pineapple, chopped
- 3 tsp. amber agave nectar (optional)
- 2 Tbs. dried, shredded coconut

Cut pineapple first and set aside one cup. Run remaining pineapple and core, through juicer, if necessary add water to equal the 2 cups needed. Or place remaining pineapple and core in high powered blender with water, strain and set aside.

Place juice, agar and agave in sauce pan (add agave only if pineapple is not sweet enough on its own). Heat on medium high, stirring often. It is acceptable to boil the mixture. It is critical to dissolve the agar completely. Add cut pineapple, cook 3 – 5 minutes. Pour into mold or dish of choice, sprinkle with coconut. Refrigerate to speed up setting process, 35 – 45 minutes.

Vanilla Coconut Ice Cream ⓟ

Recipe by Kelly Marra, RawLifeCoaching.com
Makes ¾ quart

1 cup Thai coconut meat, tightly packed

2 cups Thai coconut water

½ cups amber agave nectar or honey

1 cup raw cashews

3 – 4 vanilla beans or 1 ½ tsp. alcohol-free vanilla extract

1 very small dash of salt

Put all ingredients in a high speed blender. Blend until thoroughly mixed. Dip a spoon into the mixture, when the spoon comes out covered in air bubbles the mixture has reached the right consistency.

Pour ice cream mixture into a prepared ice cream maker and follow the ice cream maker's instructions.

Thai Coconuts, sometimes called Sweet Young Coconuts, can be found in the refrigerated produce section of some grocery stores, health food stores and Asian supermarkets. They contain soft meat that can be pulled out with a spoon and a lot of fresh coconut water. For this recipe, buy at least 4 coconuts; it's a pain to have to go back to the store if there isn't enough meat. If the coconut meat looks very pink or purple, don't use it. The meat should be white.

Berry Coulis (M)

Makes 2 cups

1 cup fresh raspberries, plus a few for garnish

1 cup fresh blackberries, plus a few for garnishes,

¼ cup amber agave nectar

juice of ½ lemon

This is a great sauce to pour over a bowl of fruit. Mix berries, sweetener, and lemon juice in a small saucepan. Simmer approximately 20 minutes on low. Remove from heat. Mash berries slightly and chill.

Brown Rice Tortilla Chips (P)

Each tortilla makes 12 chips

8-inch brown rice tortilla

olive oil

seasonings of choice, such as dried basil, rosemary, thyme, sea salt, etc

Great with the Avocado Dip from the Dressings, Sauces & Dips section.

Preheat oven to 350°. Brush both sides of tortillas lightly with olive oil. Sprinkle with seasonings. Using a sharp pair of scissors, or pizza slicer cut tortilla into 12 triangles. Lay loosely on cookie sheet, do not over lap. Bake 10 minutes until lightly browned. Watch closely to prevent burning. Let cool.

21-Day Meal Plan

21-Day Meal Plan

Making the switch to a new way of eating can be a little daunting. So I've created a 21-Day Meal Plan to guide you in the early weeks. You can follow this plan exactly as is or substitute similar dishes to better suit your personal preference. When you've complete the 21 Days you should be ready to start creating your own meal plans, but you can also simply start over and work through the plan again.

General Mealtime Guidelines

- Start your day with a glass of pure water. Add some fresh lemon juice.
- Always eat raw before cooked and wait at least 20 minutes to consume cooked.
- 75% of your daily intake should be vegetables and some fruit.
- Eat small meals and snacks; avoid 3 large meals.
- Do not drink with meals to avoid diluting digestive enzymes. Drink before meals.
- Do not eat after 8 p.m.
- Salad everyday either as a main dish or accompanying a meal.
- Have snacks with you at all times.
- Smoothies are stand-alone meals as well as great snacks.
- Breakfast meals are not limited to breakfast type foods.

- Keep animal foods to 12 oz per week.
- "Time consuming", that is the most common, negative feedback I receive about the programs. It's not because the food takes any longer to prepare but rather because there is a learning curve in what to prepare. We all default to familiarity and ease but too often that does not fit into the program guidelines nor are these defaults in your best interest. For working moms and busy business folks, planning will be the key to a successful meal time. So here are some planning tips:
- Smoothies are perfect for getting in those extra veggies. They make a great stand-alone breakfast. Make a enough for breakfast and extra for 1 or 2 snacks.
- Make a smaller smoothie when having other foods for breakfast but still make extra for snack time. Best to fill the container to the very top to keep out as much air as possible. Any smoothie can be made with 1 cup of liquid, 6-8 oz of greens and 1 cup of fruit.
- Set aside a block of time on a set day each week and cook several meals for the upcoming week.
- Double or triple all meals that are freezable. This provides those fast dinners for the following week and cuts down on cooking time.
- Make a triple batch of Cauliflower Soup Base. Make 2 Creamy Cauliflower Soups one for dinner and freeze the other. Also freeze the third batch of soup base to make Fish Chowder later.
- Make a triple batch of Vegetable Broth and follow the same premise above with Vegetable Brown Rice Soup, Roasted Vegetable Soup and Green Life Minestrone Soup.
- Make a very, very large batch of Roasted Root Vegetables or other vegetables. Use for multiple meals over a few days. Serve one night with a salad, put leftovers on your salad for lunch the next day and

make Roasted Vegetable Soup or top a gluten-free pizza.

- Make extra batches of the grain dishes (like Versatile Southwestern Rice) one for supper, top a salad the next day for lunch, put leftovers in broth the next night for soup with a salad.
- Lunch: salads, bowl of steamed vegetables with a dressing, leftovers, soup.
- Make extra bean salads and mix with rice or top salads for lunches for the next few days.

Day One

Breakfast	*Snack*	*Lunch*	*Snack*	*Dinner*
16 oz Creamy Peach Smoothie *Make extra for snack*	1 Almond Flour Muffin with caffeine free tea or almond milk	Cuc-Zuc Salad	Smoothie from breakfast	Roasted Root Vegetables with green salad

Day Two

Breakfast	*Snack*	*Lunch*	*Snack*	*Dinner*
Pear Crisp and Zippy I Smoothie *Make extra crisp for tomorrow* *Make 2 extra 8 oz smoothies for snacks*	Zippy I Smoothie	Leftover Roasted Root Vegetables on top of a bed of greens with fresh lemon	Zippy I Smoothie	Grilled Cilantro Chicken with steamed broccoli

Day Three

Breakfast	*Snack*	*Lunch*	*Snack*	*Dinner*
Pear Crisp leftovers and 8 oz Apple Pie Smoothie *Make extra smoothie for snack*	1 Almond Flour Muffin with caffeine free tea or almond milk	Marinated Bean Salad. *Make extra for tomorrow*	Apple Pie Smoothie	Roasted Vegetable Soup using leftovers from Roasted Root Vegetables

Day Four

Breakfast	*Snack*	*Lunch*	*Snack*	*Dinner*
8 oz Green Power Smoothie *Make extra for snack* Swiss Chard Pie *Make extra for lunch (eat with a salad), dinner (eat with a salad and/ or vegetable) or breakfast tomorrow*	1 - 2 cups fresh snap peas with 1 oz sheep feta	Leftover Marinated Bean Salad on top of a bed of greens	Green Power Smoothie	Versatile Southwestern Rice *Make extra for Day 6 lunch and soup tomorrow*

Day Five

Breakfast	*Snack*	*Lunch*	*Snack*	*Dinner*
8 oz Bob's Very Berry Beet Smoothie with oatmeal *Make extra smoothie for snack*	Fresh vegetables with a Bean Dip *Make extra for the next few days*	Leftover Swiss Chard Pie with green salad	Bob's Very Berry Beet Smoothie	Add leftover Versatile Southwestern Rice to broth for soup, with green salad

Day Six

Breakfast	*Snack*	*Lunch*	*Snack*	*Dinner*
16 oz Vegetable Smoothie *Make extra for snack*	Celery with raw nut butter	Cheesy Cauliflower *Use a small head and eat it all!*	Vegetable Smoothie	Leftover Versatile Southwestern Rice on top of a bed of greens with lemon juice

Day Seven

Start to think about the individual foods that are part of the program and are foods that you enjoy. Even though they are not a recipe in this book, use your imagination and information you have learned to create your own choices, such as oatmeal, hot rice or quinoa cereal or even eggs for breakfast.

When creating your own ideas, simply follow the guidelines of the program. Hard boiled eggs or omelets with vegetables are great. For smoothies, blend fruit, liquid and greens according to your taste buds and desires; add cinnamon or nutmeg. For lunch or dinner, incorporate your favorite recipes but modify them according to the program guidelines; try rice tortilla pizzas and salads of your own creation!

Breakfast	*Snack*	*Lunch*	*Snack*	*Dinner*
Rolled Oats Hot Cereal *Make smoothies for both snacks.*	Smoothie you made in the morning	Big salad of greens, sliced apple, sliced almonds, chopped celery and top with Apple Nut Butter Dressing *Make extra salad to have with dinner*	Smoothie you made in the morning	Salad from lunch with Grilled Cilantro Chicken and steamed asparagus *Grill extra chicken and freeze it for chicken salad later in the week or add it to a soup*

Day Eight

Breakfast	*Snack*	*Lunch*	*Snack*	*Dinner*
Arugula Frittata	Rice crackers with mashed avocado	Kale Salad *Make extra for tomorrow*	Smoothie from breakfast	Bean Chili and Sweet Potato with a salad *You guessed it, make extra for tomorrow!*

Day Nine

Breakfast	*Snack*	*Lunch*	*Snack*	*Dinner*
Smoothie of your choice *Make extra for snack*	Fruit salad drizzled with Almond Nut Butter Dressing *Makes a great breakfast too! Cut extra fruit for tomorrow*	Leftover Kale Salad	Smoothie from breakfast	Leftover Bean Chili and Sweet Potato with a salad

Day Ten

Breakfast	*Snack*	*Lunch*	*Snack*	*Dinner*
Big bowl of fruit you cut for yesterday's snack Sprinkle with chopped nuts and cinnamon	Almond Flour Muffin (Remember they are frozen, so allow time for defrosting)	Green Rice *Make extra for tomorrow*	Keep frozen vegetables on hand for quick, easy lunches and snacks Top with lemon juice and sheep or goat feta	Pasta with Fresh Avocado Sauce

Day Eleven

Breakfast	*Snack*	*Lunch*	*Snack*	*Dinner*
Green Power Smoothie *Make extra for snack*	Chopped celery and apple with raw nut butter	Leftover Green Rice	Smoothie from breakfast	Creamy Cauliflower Soup with a green salad *Make extra and freeze one or two batches for soup next week*

Day Twelve

Breakfast	*Snack*	*Lunch*	*Snack*	*Dinner*
One apple or pear Wait 20 minutes to eat Gluten Free Pancakes	1 cup raw snap peas	Raw celery and or carrot sticks plain or dipped in Artichoke Sunflower Spread	Smoothie from breakfast	Hearty Vegetable Soup *Make extra and freeze for Day 17*

Day Thirteen

Breakfast	*Snack*	*Lunch*	*Snack*	*Dinner*
Smoothie of your choice *Make extra for snack*	Almond Flour Muffin	Broccoli Apple Salad *Make extra for tomorrow*	Smoothie from breakfast	White Bean Chili with a green salad *Make extra for tomorrow*

Day Fourteen

Breakfast	*Snack*	*Lunch*	*Snack*	*Dinner*
Creamy Peach Smoothie *Make extra for snack*	Stuffed Apple *Make several (they also make a tasty breakfast)*	Leftover Broccoli Apple Salad	Smoothie from breakfast	Leftover White Bean Chili with a green salad

Day Fifteen

Breakfast	*Snack*	*Lunch*	*Snack*	*Dinner*
Piece of fruit then wait 20 minutes before eating hot oatmeal, rice or quinoa cereal *Make Zippie I Smoothie for snack while cereal is cooking*	Nut Butter Wraps	Crunchy Salad	Smoothie from breakfast	Steak Salad

Day Sixteen

Breakfast	*Snack*	*Lunch*	*Snack*	*Dinner*
Swiss Chard Pie *Make extra for tomorrow morning*	Stuffed Apple	Asian Grain *Make extra for Day 18*	Smoothie from breakfast	Fish Chowder with green salad *Use the frozen Cauliflower Soup Base*

Day Seventeen

Breakfast	*Snack*	*Lunch*	*Snack*	*Dinner*
Leftover Swiss Chard Pie *Make Green Power Smoothie for both snacks*	Smoothie from the morning	Any chopped greens topped with a Marinated Bean Salad	Smoothie from the morning	Medi-terranean Vegetable Pizza Serve with a side salad *Make Baked Brown Rice Pudding for tomorrow and Day 19*

Day Eighteen

Breakfast	*Snack*	*Lunch*	*Snack*	*Dinner*
Baked Brown Rice Pudding that you made yesterday	Fruit with nuts or nut butter	Leftover Asian Grain from Day 16	Stuffed Apple *Make extra for breakfast and snacks for upcoming days*	Garlicky Beans and Greens with a green salad *Make a double batch to use tomorrow.*

Day Nineteen

Breakfast	*Snack*	*Lunch*	*Snack*	*Dinner*
Fruit and Nutty Smoothie *Make extra for the afternoon snack*	Baked Brown Rice Pudding	Veggie Wraps	Smoothie from breakfast	Garlicky Beans and Greens soup made from last night's leftovers and broth.

Day Twenty

Breakfast	*Snack*	*Lunch*	*Snack*	*Dinner*
Apple Pie Smoothie *Make extra for afternoon snack*	Fruit & Oat Cobbler *Make extra for breakfast tomorrow*	Spinach and Asian Pear Salad	Smoothie from breakfast	Craig's Honduras Chicken, Faux-tatoes and green salad *Make chicken broth from bones & reserve leftover chicken for tomorrow and next week*

Day Twenty-One

Breakfast	*Snack*	*Lunch*	*Snack*	*Dinner*
Fruit & Oat Cobbler	Rice crackers with mashed avocado	Chicken Salad *Use the leftover chicken from last night*	Raw vegetables dipped in Artichoke Sauce/Dip *Make extra sauce to use for on pasta or for dipping more vegetables for snack tomorrow*	Kickin' Black Bean Soup with green salad. *Don't forget those extras for tomorrow!*

Congratulations! You completed the 21 days and now have a clear understanding on how to plan your meals. If you don't feel like you are ready to go it on your own then start the 21 days over until you feel comfortable. You can also follow the 21 day plan and simply put in other recipes to best suit your preference.

here's to our health!

Index

Index

A

Acknowledgements 11
adzuki beans 74
Agar Agar 182, 200, 201
agave nectar, amber 199, 200, 201, 202, 203
alfalfa sprouts 24
almond butter 158, 172, 197
almond flour 61, 184, 194
Almond Flour Muffins 184
almond milk 133, 134, 138, 140, 146, 154, 156, 158, 162, 171, 191
almonds 165, 195, 199, 200
aloe vera 174
amaranth 48
Ap-a-cado (with Dates) Smoothie 171
Apple Bread(less) Pudding 198
Apple-Cado Smoothie 171
apple juice 194
Apple Nut Butter Dressing 158
Apple Nut Milk 175
Apple Pie Smoothie 171
apples 37, 61, 115, 117, 121, 122, 140, 158, 171, 172, 173, 174, 175, 177, 184, 188, 192, 193, 196, 197, 198
Apple Tahini Dressing 158
arrowroot powder 190, 194
artichoke hearts 24, 57, 77, 89, 100, 105, 110, 119, 122, 124, 126, 160, 161, 162, 164
Artichoke Sauce/Dip 160
Artichoke Sunflower Spread 161
arugula 24, 44, 53, 143
Arugula Fritata 44
Arugula Frittata 44
Asian Grain 49
asparagus 26, 40, 52, 113, 120, 121, 141
avocado 49, 55, 58, 78, 98, 108, 113, 114, 122, 154, 156, 159, 160, 161, 162, 171, 173, 174
Avocado Pesto Stuffed Cucumber 108
Avocado Sauce/Dip 162
Avo-Choke Sauce/Dip 162

B

Baked Apple Fennel 37
Baked Brown Rice Pudding 190
Baked Fish Florentine 100
Baked Fruit Bowl 192
Baked Peaches with Nut Cream 191
Baked Spaghetti Squash 31
baking powder 59, 60, 61, 81, 184, 185, 186, 198
baking soda 60
bananas 200
basil 32, 41, 53, 54, 55, 58, 77, 78, 88, 92, 108, 109, 114, 136, 144, 160, 162, 163, 164
basil pesto 33
Basil Pesto 164
bay leaf 67, 91, 135, 144
Bean Chili and Sweet Potatoes 74
Bean Dips 79
beans 63
  adzuki 74
  black 66, 68, 74, 75, 78, 80, 81
  black eyed peas 66, 78
  cannelli 66, 79
  cannellini 66, 67, 69, 70, 71, 79
  chickpeas 66
  common types 66
  great northern 67
  green 24, 138, 144
  kidney 66
  lima 66
  navy 69
  pinto 66
  preparation tips 66
  string 26, 127
  white 66, 67, 69, 70, 73, 77, 79, 80
  white kidney 74
Bean Salads, Marinated 77
Beans Chapter 63
beef 145
  ground 95
beets 116, 172
Beet Salad 116
bell peppers 35, 68
  red 68
  roasted 79
berries 157
Berry Coulis 203
Berrylicious Dressing 157
Beverages 170
Black Bean and Corn Salad 78
Black Bean Dip, Spicy 80
black beans 66, 68, 74, 75, 78, 80, 81
blackberries 203
Black Eyed Pea and Cucumber Salad 78
black eyed peas 66, 78
black pepper 27, 71, 93, 135
blueberries 172
Bob's Very Berry Beet Smoothie 172
Braggs 112
broccoli 26, 30, 117, 136, 139, 146
  florets 122, 136
  stalk 122
  stems 136
Broccoli Apple Salad 117
broth 134, 138, 139, 144, 163

chicken 67, 69, 70, 73, 136, 137, 138, 140, 141, 142, 143, 145
vegetable 68, 100, 136, 138, 141
brown rice 48, 49, 50, 51, 52, 53, 54, 56, 75, 118, 138, 141, 174, 175, 189, 190
brown rice flour 59, 60, 164, 186
brown rice pasta 58
brown rice tortilla 203
Brown Rice Tortilla Chips 203
Brown Rice with Asparagus 52
brussels sprouts 24, 26, 30
Bryn, Dotty 32
buckwheat 48, 174
butter 59
Butternut Squash 31
Butternut Squash Soup 140

C

cabbage 26, 30, 50, 56, 95, 112, 115, 122, 136, 138, 144
bok choy 24
cannellini beans 66, 67, 69, 70, 71, 79
capers 80
Caramelized Brown Rice Pudding 189
cardamom 192
carrots 25, 26, 30, 49, 50, 51, 68, 70, 80, 92, 93, 112, 115, 118, 121, 122, 126, 127, 134, 135, 138, 144, 145, 146, 163, 172, 188
cashew butter 158
Cashew Cream 187
cashews 133, 138, 155, 157, 159, 165, 187, 202
cauliflower 24, 26, 30, 37, 38, 39, 133, 134, 146, 163
Cauliflower Soup Base 133
cayenne 68
celeriac 38, 135
Celeriac Sauté 38
celery 24, 38, 70, 77, 78, 92, 93, 105, 113, 120, 122, 124, 139, 145, 146, 173
celery leaves 38
chard 71
cheese
feta 77, 78, 89, 93, 106, 116, 119, 124
goat 32, 39, 43, 105, 109
Pecorino Romano 39, 71, 75, 77
sheep 32, 43, 105, 109
Cheesy Cauliflower 39
chia seed 174
chicken 121, 126, 145
breast 87, 89, 92, 94, 144
cutlets 88
shredded 95
whole 90, 91
chicken broth 67, 69, 70, 73, 136, 137, 138, 140, 141, 142, 143, 145
Chicken Salad 126
chicken sausage 143
Chicken Sausage Soup 143
chickpeas 66
chili pepper 68
green 73, 75
chili powder 73, 74
chives 126
chocolate chips 81
chopped tomatoes 70, 74
cilantro 52, 55, 57, 68, 74, 75, 78, 80, 87, 111, 113, 114, 126, 154, 161, 165
Cilantro Pesto 165
cinnamon 171, 175, 176, 187, 188, 189, 190, 192, 193, 194, 197, 198
sticks 195
cloves 195
cocoa nibs 81
cocoa powder 81
coconut 201, 202
coconut milk 190, 200
coconut oil 81, 185, 186, 192
coconut water 155, 202
Cold Rice Noodle Salad 57
collard greens 24, 44, 56, 95, 142
Collard Greens Minera 44
coriander 80
corn 73, 78
Craig's Honduras Chicken 90
cranberry juice 195
Creamed Kale 42
Creamy Avocado and Herb Dressing 156
Creamy Carrot Soup 138
Creamy Cauliflower Soup 134
Creamy Herb Dressing 154
Creamy Lemony Dressing 156
Creamy Peach Smoothie 172
Creamy White Bean Soup 67
Crispy Sugar Snap Pea Salad 111
Crunchy Salad 124
cucumber 24, 49, 52, 107, 120, 121, 126, 154, 158, 159, 173, 178
English 52, 55, 57, 78, 99, 105, 106, 108, 109, 110, 111, 114, 119, 122, 124, 126, 154, 158, 174
Cucumber Dressing 154
Cuc-Zuc 109
cumin 68, 73, 74, 78, 80

D

Dairy-free Cream Soups 132
dates 171, 187, 198, 199, 200
dill 97, 98, 99, 106, 107, 154, 159
Dressings, Sauces, & Dips Chapter 149

E

Easy Crockpot Chicken or Turkey 92

edamame 51, 118
eggs 43, 44, 59, 61, 184, 185, 186, 189
egg whites 198
endive 24
English Cucumber Salad 105
escarole 24, 41, 69, 70, 143

F

fennel 24, 26, 30, 36, 37, 53, 92, 136
bulb 144, 145
Fennel 36
fennel seed 37, 80, 93, 95, 142, 143
fish
salmon 97, 98, 146
tuna 99
white 100, 146
Fish Chowder 146
flour
almond 61, 184, 194
brown rice 59, 60, 164, 186
oat 198
quinoa 185
tapioca 185
tapioca starch 59, 60
Fresh Cucumber Dip 159
frittata 44
Fruit Kabobs 192
Fruit & Nutty Smoothie 172
Fruit & Oat Cobbler 193
Fruit Pie, 20 Minute 199
Fruity Iced Tea Cooler 177

G

garlic 26, 30, 35, 39, 41, 50, 54, 56, 67, 68, 69, 70, 71, 78, 79, 80, 87, 90, 92, 93, 94, 95, 98, 100, 107, 108, 116, 127, 133, 135, 138, 139, 141, 142, 143, 145, 154, 155, 156, 157, 159, 160, 161, 163, 164, 165, 166
Garlicky Beans and Greens 71
Garlicky Lemon Dressing 155
garlic powder 67, 97
ginger 90, 138
Gluten-Free Pancakes 60
Grains Chapter 45
granola 191, 193
Granola, Homemade 186
grapefruit 178
Grated Carrot 115
great northern beans 67
Greek Cucumber 106
green beans 24, 39, 122, 136, 138, 144
Green Life Minestrone 141
green onion 113
Green Power Smoothie 173
Green Rice 54
greens 172, 173, 174
mixed 53
Greens and Turkey Bacon 142
Green Velvet Dressing/Dip 159
Grilled Chicken with Gourmet Herb Sauce 88
Grilled Cilantro Chicken 87
Grilled Romaine 125
Grilled Salmon and Zucchini 97
Grilled Salmon with Avocado Dip 98
Grilled Vegetables 29
Grilled Vegetables with Rice 53
Grilled Yellow Fin Tuna 99

H

Harris, Amanda 146
hazelnuts 81
hearts of palm 120
Hearts of Palm 120
Hearty Vegetable Soup 136
hemp seed 60
Herbed Chicken Salad 126
Hijiki 51, 118
Hijiki Seaweed Rollup 118
Hijiki with Rice 51
honey 90, 198, 202
'Hot' Oatmeal Smoothie 175
hot sauce 78, 80

I

Italian White Bean Soup 70

K

Kabobs 94
kale 24, 42, 113, 142, 143, 144, 172
Kale Salad 112
Kickin' Black Bean Soup 68
kidney beans 66
Kob Farms House Dressing 155
kohlrabi 24, 36, 92
Kohlrabi 36

L

leek 69, 70, 71
lemon 27, 31, 36, 37, 39, 40, 41, 44, 50, 51, 52, 53, 54, 55, 56, 57, 58, 78, 89, 94, 95, 120, 127, 146, 160, 162, 198
juice 77, 79, 80, 88, 97, 98, 100, 107, 108, 110, 111, 113, 114, 115, 116, 117, 118, 119, 120, 125, 126, 127, 136, 154, 155, 156, 157, 159, 160, 162, 164, 165, 173, 174, 194, 199, 203
zest 98, 100, 155, 156, 157
Lemony Nutty Green Beans 39
lettuce 126
escarole 24, 41, 69, 70, 143
romaine 24, 41, 125, 126, 127, 173, 174, 188
Light Raisin Dressing 158
lima beans 66
lime 31, 36, 44, 52, 53, 75, 87, 99, 126
juice 49, 105, 109, 124, 161

M

macadamia nuts 156, 159, 165
mango 200
maple syrup 81, 190, 194, 198
marjoram 35, 92
Marra, Kelly 199
Meal Plan, 21-Day 205
meatballs 145
Meatball Vegetable Soup 145
Meats Chapter 83
  unclean 86
Mediterranean Vegetable Pizza 35
milk
  almond 133, 134, 138, 140, 146, 154, 156, 158, 162, 171, 191
  coconut 190, 200
  nut 42, 61
  rice 42, 61, 154, 156, 158, 164, 171, 185, 186, 189
millet 174
mint 52, 55, 56, 95, 107, 124, 126, 165, 174
Mint Pesto 165
Mock Fried Rice 50
mustard
  stone-ground 155
mustard greens 24

N

navy beans 69
Nori 49, 118
nut butter 121, 188, 191
Nut Butter Wraps 188
nutmeg 176, 187, 189, 192, 193, 194, 197, 198
Nut Milk, Homemade 175
Nutnog/Seednog 176
nuts 39, 42, 61, 115, 144, 175, 176, 186, 191, 192, 196, 197
Nutty Dippin' 188

O

oat flour 198
oats 48, 174, 175, 186, 197, 198
  quick 81
  rolled 61
oil 194
okra 24, 28
olive oil 27, 28, 31, 32, 34, 36, 37, 39, 41, 53, 54, 61, 67, 69, 70, 71, 99, 105, 106, 109, 110, 112, 116, 118, 119, 120, 125, 134, 144, 155, 156, 159, 161, 164, 165, 166, 186, 203
Olive Pate 166
olives 35
  black 73, 75, 77, 78, 120, 124, 166
  Black 105
  green 77
  kalamata 80
  Kalamata 78, 109, 119, 166
olive tapenade 32
onion 26, 27, 35, 43, 50, 56, 67, 68, 73, 77, 93, 100, 116, 127, 138, 142, 146
  green 113
  red 92
onion flakes 42
Orange Creamsicle 177
oranges 157, 177, 195
oregano 35, 53, 55, 68, 73, 88, 89, 93, 94, 106, 120, 124, 135, 136, 145, 161

P

parsley 27, 39, 54, 56, 88, 92, 93, 95, 119, 124, 126, 135, 136, 145, 146, 159, 160, 163, 166, 173, 174
parsnips 27, 135
pasta
  brown rice 58
  rice 57
  rice noodles 57
Pasta Sauce 163
Pasta with Fresh Avocado Sauce 58
peaches 61, 122, 172, 174, 175, 176, 177, 191, 192, 193
Peach Nut Milk 176
Pea-Cumber 110
Pear-Apple Sauce 196
Pear Crisp 194
pears 61, 121, 122, 173, 174, 175, 177, 192, 193, 194, 195, 196
  Asian 117
peas 50, 55, 57, 105, 110, 119, 122, 136, 141, 145
  green 55
  snow 24, 141
  sugar snap 24, 111, 122, 141
Peas and Lettuce 41
pecans 195
pepitas 174
pepper
  bell 35, 68
  black 27
  cayenne 68
  chile 68
pineapple 200, 201
Pineapple Coconut Not-Jello 201
pineapple juice 201
pine nuts 108, 155, 156, 159, 164, 165, 166
pinto beans 66
Poached Pears 195
Prescription for Wellness 13
pumpkin seeds 32, 113, 174
pumpkin spice 187

Q

quinoa 48, 49, 174, 185
quinoa flour 185

R

radishes 24
  daikon 51, 118
  red 111
raisins 158, 189, 190
raspberries 203
Raw Asparagus & Kale "Guacamole" Salad 113
red leaf (greens) 24
Reece, Glenda 138
rice 55
  brown 48, 49, 50, 51, 52, 53, 54, 56, 75, 118, 138, 141, 174, 175, 189, 190
  wild 48
Rice Flour Muffins 186
rice milk 42, 61, 154, 156, 158, 164, 171, 185, 186, 189
rice noodles 57
rice pasta 48, 57
Rice Stuffed Cabbage Leaves 56
Roasted Root Vegetables 27
roasted vegetables 137
Roasted Vegetable Soup 137
Roasted Whole Okra 28
romaine lettuce 24, 41, 125, 126, 127, 173, 174, 188
rosemary 53, 67, 70, 79, 80, 89, 92, 94, 114, 135
Ruby Red Cucumber 178
rutabaga 24

S

sage 79
Salads Chapter 101
salsa 74, 75
salt 60, 61, 155, 161, 184, 202
  sea salt 27, 59, 81, 113, 185, 190, 194, 198
Sans Cream of Broccoli 139
Sautéed Escarole 41
scallions 67, 71, 73, 74, 78, 142
seaweeds 49
  Nori 49
sesame oil 49, 50, 51, 57, 118
sesame seeds 49, 111, 158
  black 50, 57
sherry 90
Smoothies 170
Smoothies & Beverages Chapter 167
snow peas 24, 141
Soups Chapter 129
Spaghetti Squash 32
Spaghetti Squash "Pasta" 33
Speedy Vegetable Soup 136
spinach 51, 53, 54, 89, 93, 95, 100, 117, 118, 119, 127, 136, 140, 143, 144, 161, 171, 173
Spinach and Asian Pear Salad 117
sprouts 24
  alfalfa 24
  brussel 24, 26, 30
squash
  butternut 26, 30, 140
  spaghetti 31, 32, 33
  summer 24, 25, 26, 30, 53
  winter 27
  yellow 119, 121, 122, 163
  zucchini 24, 25, 26, 30, 34, 35, 53, 54, 55, 56, 93, 95, 97, 109, 121, 122, 136, 144, 145, 163
Squash-n-Hearts 119
steak 127
Steak Salad 127
Steamed Pea Pods 40
strawberries 200
string beans 26, 127
Stuffed Avocado 114
sugar snap peas 24, 40, 111, 122, 141
sunflower butter 154
sunflower seeds 161
Sunshine Dressing 157
Super Healthy Guacamole Dip 161
Super Smoothie 174
sweet potatoes 27, 59, 74, 78
Sweet Potato (or Yam) Biscuits 59
Sweet Slaw 115
swiss chard 43, 142, 143
  stalks 43
Swiss Chard Pie 43

T

tahini 158, 159, 173
Tangy Cashew Dressing 157
tapioca 185
tapioca flour 185
tapioca starch 59, 60
tarragon 42, 88, 120, 126, 136, 159
tea, caffeine free 177
teff 48
thyme 35, 41, 53, 92, 127, 139, 144
tomatoes 78
  cherry 70
  chopped 70, 74
  diced 68
  fresh 75
  grape 67
  sun dried 67, 77, 78, 79, 80
  sundried 67
tortilla, brown rice 203
Treats Chapter 179
Tropical Panna Cotta Pie 200
turkey 121
  breast 92
  ground 93, 95
turkey bacon 44, 142
Turkey Meatloaf 93
turnip greens 24
turnips 24, 27

V

vanilla 81, 158, 171, 175, 176, 186, 187, 189, 190, 191, 194, 202
  bean 175, 176, 177, 202
Vanilla Coconut Ice Cream 202
vegetable broth 68, 100, 136, 138, 141

Vegetable Broth, Homemade 135
Vegetable Brown Rice Soup 138
Vegetable Chicken Soup 144
Vegetable Kabobs 30
Vegetables Chapter 23
Vegetable Smoothie 173
Veggie Master Mixes 122
Veggie Wraps 121
Versatile Southwestern Rice 75
vinegar 77, 157
  apple cider, raw 54, 112
  balsamic 27
  Riesling Raisin 158

W

walnuts 37, 81, 115, 117, 171, 193, 195, 198, 200
water chestnuts 24
watercress 24, 119
Watercress Salad 119
White Bean and Roasted Pepper Dip 79
White Bean and Sun Dried Tomato Dip 79
White Bean Artichoke Salad 77
White Bean Chili 73
white beans 66, 67, 69, 70, 73, 77, 79, 80
White Bean "Tapenade" 80
White Bean with Escarole Soup 69
white kidney beans 74
White Sauce 164
Willix, Bob 172
wine
  white 90

X

xanthan gum 59

Y

yams 59
yogurt
  goat 88, 98, 107

Z

Zesty Asparagus 40
Zippy Smoothie I 173
Zippy Smoothie II 174
Zucchini Rollups 34

About the Author

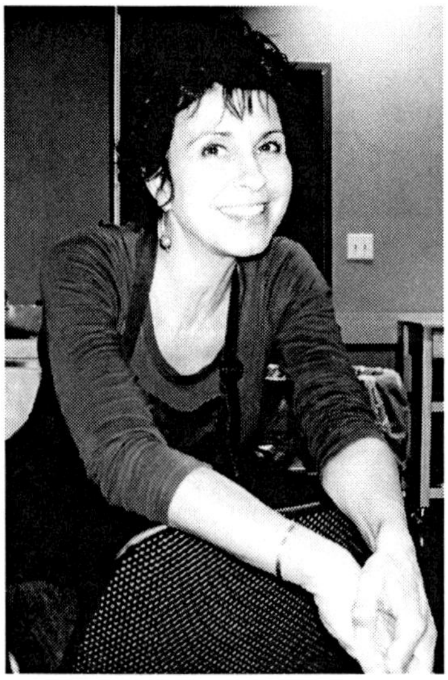

Denise Souza began her personal journey to wellness through holistic modalities and nutritious food when she was diagnosed with Gilbert Syndrome in the late 1980's. At eight years old, her daughter was misdiagnosed with migraines, constipation and far-sighted vision. During the same time, her son had chronic ear infections and respiratory congestion.

After no resolution with traditional means, Denise sought holistic answers with Dr. Stephen Driscoll. Their rapid success with holistic modalities led Denise to study this field and share her knowledge.

Denise is a mother, health advocate, holistic nutrition lifestyle consultant, colon therapist, lecturer, cancer survivor, educator, and perpetual student. She holds a Master of Science with high honors in Holistic Nutrition and a Bachelor of Art in Psychology. As a Colon Hydrotherapist she is certified by the International Association for Colon Hydrotherapy and the National Board for Colon Hydrotherapy. Denise also served as secretary of the North Carolina Colon Hydrotherapy Safety Association and vice president of the American Holistic Medical Association. She has completed Level 4 in Touch for Health training and is trained in Bio-Electrical Impedance

Measurement testing. She is co-founder and facilitator of the GET LEAN Weight Loss and Wellness Program as well as the Prescription for Wellness Program.

Denise believes we are creations of God and stands in awe at the magnificence and intricacies of the body. The workings and abilities of the body can sometimes seem so complex at times, yet the blueprint for wellness is quite simple when empowered with knowledge. Denise's goal is to teach her clients not to limit their changes or goals to a short window of time or specific short-term goal but rather to think of lifestyle changes. Through educating her clients she believes they are empowered to change their lifestyle, which in turn changes their lives. She encourages clients to think outside the box, whether modifying a recipe, reshaping their perception of nutrition, dieting, detoxifying or desiring overall wellness.

In 2006, Denise and her husband, Jerry, moved from Massachusetts to Raleigh, North Carolina. They both enjoy the outdoors and the wonderful, long summer days. They have three grown children and three grandchildren scattered around the world.

Denise can be contacted by emailing BodySymmetry@gmail.com or visiting BodySymmetry-Wellness.com.

Doctor References

Dr. John Schmitt, DC
182 Windchime Ct., Raleigh, NC, 27615
919-847-3555

Dr. Angela Baylis, DC
182 Windchime Ct., Raleigh, NC, 27615
919-417-4414

Dr. Amanda Keates, DC
182 Windchime Ct., Raleigh, NC, 27615
919-400-7909

Dr. Joanne Pizzino, MD
1350 SE Maynard Rd., Cary, NC 27511
919-651-0820

CPSIA information can be obtained at www.ICGtesting.com
Printed in the USA
BVOW062046040613

322440BV00003B/10/P

9 781611 530315